P9-DYB-630

Pathology

**PreTest®
Self-Assessment
and Review**

• NOTICE •

Medicine is an ever-changing science. As new research and clinical experience broaden our knowledge, changes in treatment and drug therapy are required. The editors and the publisher of this work have checked with sources believed to be reliable in their efforts to provide information that is complete and generally in accord with the standards accepted at the time of publication. However, in view of the possibility of human error or changes in medical sciences, neither the editor, nor the publisher, nor any other party who has been involved in the preparation or publication of this work warrants that the information contained herein is in every respect accurate or complete. Readers are encouraged to confirm the information contained herein with other sources. For example and in particular, readers are advised to check the product information sheet included in the package of each drug they plan to administer to be certain that the information contained in this book is accurate and that changes have not been made in the recommended dose or in the contraindications for administration. This recommendation is of particular importance in connection with new or infrequently used drugs.

Pathology

PreTest®
Self-Assessment
and Review

Sixth Edition

Edited by

Margaret H.S. Clements, M.D.
Visiting Professor of Pathology
Cornell University Medical College
New York, New York

With questions contributed by

Michael D. Jeffers, M.B.
Senior House Officer
St. James's Hospital
Dublin, Ireland

McGraw-Hill, Inc.
Health Professions Division/PreTest Series

New York   St. Louis   San Francisco   Colorado Springs
Auckland   Bogotá   Hamburg   Lisbon   London   Madrid
Mexico   Milan   Montreal   New Delhi   Paris   San Juan
São Paulo   Singapore   Sydney   Tokyo   Toronto

Pathology: PreTest Self-Assessment and Review

Copyright © 1991 1988 1986 1983 1980 1976 by McGraw-Hill, Inc. All rights reserved. Printed in the United States of America. Except as permitted under the Copyright Act of 1976, no part of this publication may be reproduced or distributed in any form or by any means, or stored in a data base or retrieval system, without the prior written permission of the publisher.

2 3 4 5 6 7 8 9 0   DOCDOC   9 8 7 6 5 4 3 2 1

ISBN 0-07-051975-7

This book was set in Times Roman by Waldman Graphics, Inc.
The editors were Gail Gavert and Bruce MacGregor.
The production supervisor was Clara B. Stanley.
R.R. Donnelley & Sons was printer and binder.

Library of Congress Cataloging-in-Publication Data

Pathology : PreTest self-assessment and review.—6th ed. / edited by
    Margaret H.S. Clements.
        p.   cm.
    Includes bibliographical references.
    ISBN 0-07-051975-7
    1. Pathology—Examinations, questions, etc.   I. Clements,
Margaret H.S.
    [DNLM: 1. Pathology—examination questions.   QZ 18 P297]
    RB31.P325   1991
    616.07'076—dc20
DNLM/DLC
for Library of Congress   90-5587
                                                                                   CIP

Contents

Preface

The study of pathology, a science so basic to clinical medicine, has been abbreviated sadly in many medical schools in recent years, and this at a time when explosive growth is occurring in the science. Recent advances in immunopathology, diagnosis of bacterial and viral diseases including AIDS, and detection of infectious agents such as papilloma virus in cervical dysplasia are proceeding at a tremendous rate. The sixth edition of *Pathology: PreTest® Self-Assessment and Review* includes such new subject areas as predictive values in the interpretation of laboratory data, importance of cytokines, the molecular basis of genetic and other disease processes, and molecular biology techniques as these apply to lymphoproliferative disorders and other tumors.

The medical student must feel submerged at times in the flood of information—occasionally instructors may have similar feelings. This edition is not intended to cover all new knowledge in addition to including older anatomic and clinical pathology. It is, rather, a serious attempt to present important facts about many disease processes in hopes that the student will read much further in major textbooks and journals and will receive some assistance in passing medical school, licensure, or board examinations.

Margaret H. S. Clements, M.D.

Introduction

Pathology: PreTest® Self-Assessment and Review provides medical students, as well as physicians, with a comprehensive and convenient instrument for self-assessment and review within the field of pathology. The 500 questions parallel the format and degree of difficulty of the questions contained in Part I of the National Board of Medical Examiners examinations, the Federation Licensing Examination (FLEX), and the Foreign Medical Graduate Examination in the Medical Sciences (FMGEMS).

Each question in the book is accompanied by an answer, an explanation, and specific page references to current textbooks, journal articles, or both. A bibliography, listing all the sources used, follows the last chapter.

Perhaps the most effective way to use this book is to allow yourself one minute to answer each question in a given chapter; as you proceed, indicate your answer beside each question. By following this suggestion, you will be approximating the time limits imposed by the board examinations previously mentioned.

When you finish answering the questions in a chapter, you should then spend as much time as you need verifying your answers and carefully reading the explanations. Although you should pay special attention to the explanations for the questions you answered incorrectly, you should read *every* explanation. The author of this book has designed the explanations to reinforce and supplement the information tested by the questions. If, after reading the explanations for a given chapter, you feel you need still more information about the material covered, you should consult and study the references indicated.

Pathology

PreTest® Self-Assessment and Review

General Pathology

DIRECTIONS: Each question below contains five suggested responses. Select the **one best** response to each question.

1. Which of the following provides an example of concomitant hyperplasia and hypertrophy?

(A) Uterine growth during pregnancy
(B) Left ventricular cardiac hypertrophy
(C) Enlargement of skeletal muscle in athletics
(D) Breast enlargement at puberty
(E) Cystic hyperplasia of the endometrium

2. Type I collagen is found in all the following EXCEPT

(A) tendon
(B) dermis
(C) cartilage
(D) fascia
(E) bone

3. Which group of factors is most important in the cellular pathogenesis of acute ischemia?

(A) Mitochondrial hyperplasia, lysozyme release, membrane injury
(B) Reduced ATP, increased calcium influx, membrane injury
(C) Lipid deposition, reduced protein synthesis, nuclear damage
(D) Ribosome detachment, glycolysis, nuclear damage
(E) Mitochondrial condensation, glycolysis, sodium cell loss

4. During early inflammation following margination of leukocytes, an important adhesive surface protein on leukocytes is

(A) interleukin-1 (IL-1)
(B) complement factor 5a (C5a)
(C) endothelial leukocyte adhesion molecule (ELAM-1)
(D) tumor necrosis factor (TNF)
(E) leukocyte function antigen-1 (LFA-1)

5. A very important mediator of the systemic effects of inflammation is

(A) gamma interferon (γ-IFN)
(B) beta tumor necrosis factor (β-TNF)
(C) interleukin-1 (IL-1)
(D) interleukin-2 (IL-2)
(E) interleukin-3 (IL-3)

6. Defects in chemotaxis resulting in increased susceptibility to infection are associated with all the following EXCEPT

(A) diabetes mellitus, juvenile type
(B) chronic granulomatous disease of childhood
(C) chronic renal failure of any cause
(D) Chédiak-Higashi syndrome
(E) newborn infants of normal gestation

7.   The cluster of cells in the photomicrograph below appeared in a cytologic specimen of sputum from a 57-year-old man with chest pain, hemoptysis, and a nonproductive cough of many years' duration. Which of the following is the most likely diagnosis?

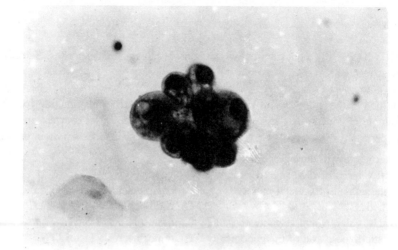

(A) Squamous cell metaplasia of ciliated, bronchial epithelium
(B) Oat cell (small-cell undifferentiated) carcinoma
(C) Adenocarcinoma
(D) Cytomegalic inclusion virus pneumonia
(E) Normal bronchial epithelium

---

8.   An understanding of complex disorders like hereditary spherocytosis, Chédiak-Higashi syndrome, and alcoholic liver disease has improved with molecular discoveries in

(A) lysosomal release
(B) recombinant DNA
(C) cytoskeletal makeup
(D) membrane phospholipids
(E) lipid accumulation

9.   Endotoxic shock is commonly caused by all the following organisms EXCEPT

(A) *Pseudomonas aeruginosa*
(B) *Escherichia coli*
(C) *Proteus* species
(D) *Corynebacterium diphtheriae*
(E) *Klebsiella pneumoniae*

10. The cells in the photomicrograph shown below are from a drop of cerebrospinal fluid. The most likely diagnosis is

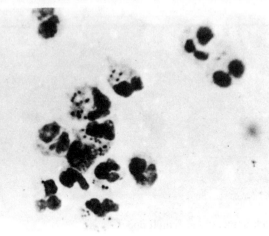

(A) subarachnoid hemorrhage
(B) viral meningitis
(C) tuberculous meningitis
(D) bacterial meningitis
(E) leukemic meningitis

---

11. The chemical mediators of inflammation listed below often proceed in a cascade after activation EXCEPT

(A) complement
(B) kinin
(C) arachidonic acid
(D) fibrinopeptides
(E) neutral proteases

12. The most common malignant neoplasm arising in the oral cavity is

(A) malignant melanoma
(B) malignant lymphoma
(C) squamous cell carcinoma
(D) necrotizing sialometaplasia
(E) Kaposi's sarcoma

13. The photomicrograph below of a duodenal aspiration smear shows an organism that

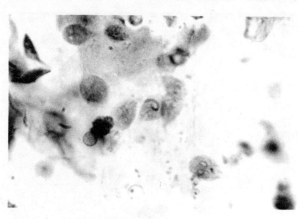

(A) is often numerous in lymph nodes
(B) infects principally the large intestine
(C) is transmitted by the genus *Triatoma*
(D) is the most common intestinal parasite in the U.S.
(E) is frequently identified in cervicovaginal smears

14. All the following characteristics are true of liposarcoma EXCEPT that it

(A) presents varied histology
(B) is commonly found in the retroperitoneum
(C) frequently gives rise to embolization in lymphatics
(D) is the most common soft tissue sarcoma
(E) arises very rarely in subcutaneous tissue

15. The cells of the mononuclear phagocyte system originate from the

(A) spleen
(B) liver
(C) lymph node
(D) bone marrow
(E) thymus

16. The histologic pattern of the lymph node section shown below is likely to support a diagnosis of

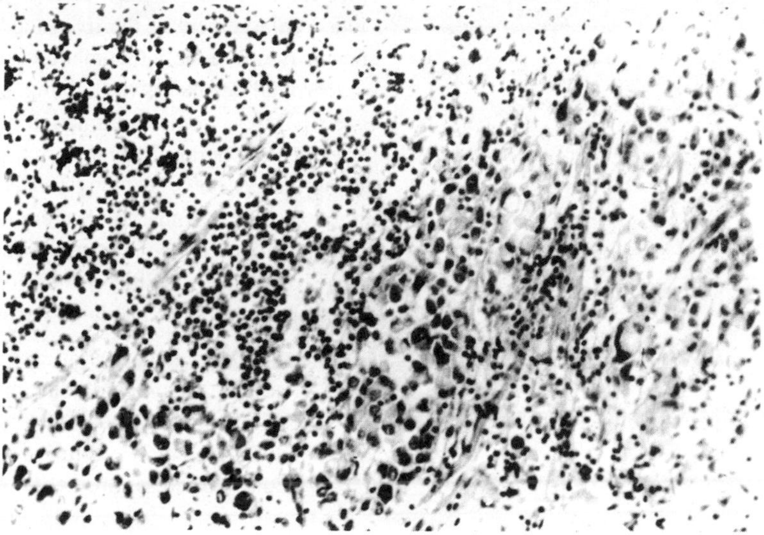

(A) sickle cell anemia
(B) carcinoma
(C) leukemia
(D) infectious mononucleosis
(E) rheumatoid arthritis

---

17. In tissues affected by the predominant form of Niemann-Pick disease, which of the following is found at abnormally high levels?

(A) Sphingomyelin
(B) Sphingomyelinase
(C) Kerasin
(D) Acetyl coenzyme A
(E) Ganglioside

18. The diseases of the Hand-Schüller-Christian complex all involve the

(A) skeleton
(B) reticuloendothelial system
(C) heart
(D) lungs
(E) teeth and nails

19. Fibrosarcoma, shown in the photomicrograph below, may be characterized by all the following EXCEPT

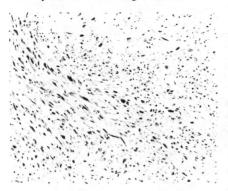

(A) interlacing bundles of anaplastic spindle cells
(B) occasional similarity to "cellular fibroma"
(C) fibroblastic or myofibroblastic differentiation
(D) relative infrequency of occurrence
(E) association with hyperglycemia

20. All the following symptoms are associated with Klinefelter's syndrome EXCEPT

(A) large, soft testes
(B) gynecomastia
(C) eunuchoidism
(D) azospermia
(E) elevated urinary gonadotropins

21. If a mutant gene is not expressed phenotypically in a person, this is said to represent

(A) variable expressivity
(B) reduced penetrance
(C) codominance
(D) genetic heterogeneity
(E) nondisjunction

22. In an evaluation of an 8-year-old boy who had had recurrent infections since the first year of life, findings included enlargement of the liver and spleen, lymph node inflammation, and a superficial dermatitis resembling eczema. Microscopic examination of a series of peripheral blood smears taken during the course of a staphylococcal infection indicated that the bactericidal capacity of the boy's neutrophils was impaired or absent. Which of the following is the most probable diagnosis?

(A) Chronic granulomatous disease
(B) Congenital agammaglobulinemia
(C) Hereditary thymic dysplasia
(D) Chédiak-Higashi syndrome
(E) Wiskott-Aldrich syndrome

23. The autosomal recessive genetic disorders known as Fanconi's anemia, ataxia telangiectasia, and Bloom's syndrome are sometimes referred to as "chromosome-breakage syndromes." The reason for this is

(A) that they are associated with leukemia
(B) that they are autosomal recessive disorders
(C) excess chromosomal vulnerability to osmotic changes
(D) increased susceptibility to cell mutations
(E) lack of DNA repair systems

24. The irregular eosinophilic hyaline inclusions within the hepatocytoplasm shown below are

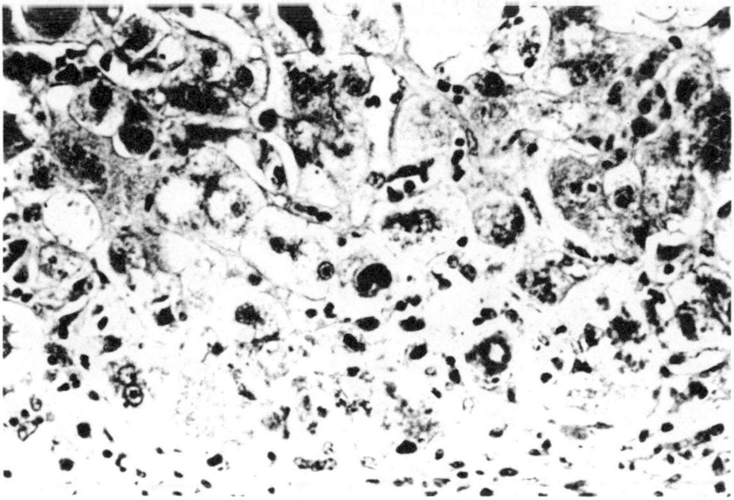

(A) Russell bodies
(B) parasites
(C) characteristic of chronic alcoholism
(D) characteristic of viral hepatitis
(E) characteristic of carbon tetrachloride poisoning

25. Interest is growing in recently discovered cell markers on neoplastic cells that are designated

(A) ADCC
(B) A1AT
(C) HIV-1
(D) TSTA
(E) ARC

26. All the following cytologic and membrane alterations can generally be found in neoplastic cells EXCEPT

(A) changes in pseudopodia and microvilli
(B) changes in the cytoskeleton
(C) acquisition of surface-associated glycoproteins
(D) increased lectin agglutinability
(E) decreased membrane transport

27. The cells seen in the following photomicrograph were stained by ABC technique using OKT1 (Leu-1), OKT3 (Leu-4), and OKT11 (Leu-5) cluster designation CD5, CD3, and CD2. The result indicates that the cells are of what origin?

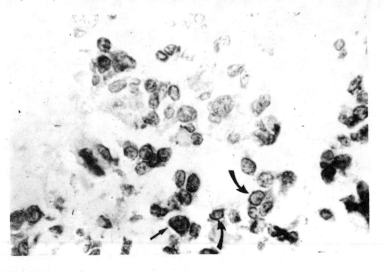

(A) T lymphocytes
(B) Oat cells
(C) Mesothelial cells
(D) EAC rosettes
(E) Melanoma cells

28. Natural killer (NK) cells have all the following characteristics EXCEPT

(A) the ability to lyse virus-infected cells
(B) cytoplasmic granules containing myeloperoxidase
(C) increased activity with stimulation by IL-2 and interferon
(D) the ability to function without prior sensitization
(E) NK receptors and Fc receptors for IgG

29. After receiving incompatible blood, a patient develops a transfusion reaction in the form of back pain, fever, shortness of breath, and hematuria. This type of immunologic reaction is classified as a

(A) systemic anaphylactic reaction
(B) systemic immune complex reaction
(C) delayed-type hypersensitivity reaction
(D) complement-mediated cytotoxicity
(E) T cell–mediated cytotoxicity

30. An industrial foundry worker who has been chronically exposed to heavy metal vapors has developed a radiographic pattern of pulmonary "honeycombing." Which of the following heavy metals is most likely responsible?

(A) Cobalt
(B) Lead
(C) Cadmium
(D) Mercury
(E) Arsenic

31. An allograft is a graft between

(A) a human and an animal
(B) two individuals of different species
(C) two individuals of the same species
(D) two individuals of the same inbred strain
(E) identical twins

32. Which of the following conditions is most likely to be associated with cancer?

(A) Systemic lupus erythematosus
(B) Hypertension
(C) Polymyositis
(D) Autoimmune thyroiditis
(E) Arteriosclerosis

33. True statements concerning diagnostic specificity include all the following EXCEPT

(A) Scl-70 antibody is specific for diffuse systemic sclerosis
(B) antibodies to nucleolar RNA are specific for diffuse systemic sclerosis
(C) antibodies to double-stranded DNA are specific for systemic lupus erythematosus (SLE)
(D) antibodies to antinuclear antibody (ANA) are specific for SLE
(E) anti-Sm antibodies are specific for SLE

34. Systemic lupus erythematosus (SLE), a multisystem disease of autoimmune origin, is characterized by all the following statements EXCEPT

(A) polyclonal B-cell activation is essential to the pathogenesis
(B) membranous glomerulonephritis is the most common renal lesion
(C) visceral lesions are mediated by type III hypersensitivity
(D) joint involvement (arthritis) is common clinically
(E) hypergammaglobulinemia is usual

35. All the following statements regarding primary Sjögren's syndrome are true EXCEPT

(A) xerostomia is a major symptom
(B) anti-SSB antibodies are major markers
(C) renal glomerular lesions are common
(D) rheumatoid factor is often present
(E) there is increased frequency of HLA-DR3

36. A patient with severe diabetic renal disease receives a donor cadaver kidney, following which a progressive rise in the serum creatinine occurs over a period lasting 5 months. In the photomicrograph below, what single finding is most characteristic for chronic rejection?

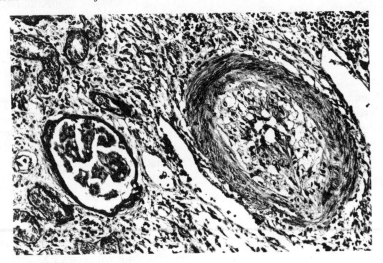

(A) Damaged glomeruli
(B) Interstitial fibrosis
(C) Interstitial inflammation
(D) Tubular atrophy
(E) Vascular changes

37. An adult patient in the summer months suffers a rash on one of the extremities followed several weeks later by arthritis of the knee. In addition to viral and bacterial disorders and rheumatoid joint disease, which of the following should also be considered in the differential diagnosis?

(A) Hemarthrosis
(B) Reiter's disease
(C) Lyme disease
(D) Charcot's joint
(E) Baker's cyst

38. Hypertrophic osteoarthropathy is most often associated with

(A) bronchiectasis
(B) infective endocarditis
(C) bronchogenic carcinoma
(D) mesothelioma
(E) inflammatory bowel disease

39. In which of the following diseases or conditions would a negative immunofluorescent procedure for detection of serum antibodies to mitochondria be expected?

(A) Primary biliary cirrhosis
(B) Chlorpromazine-induced jaundice
(C) Acute viral hepatitis
(D) Chronic active hepatitis
(E) Systemic lupus erythematosus

40. A young woman of average intelligence and short stature who has never menstruated is under clinical investigation for Turner's syndrome. However, a buccal smear shows some cells having one Barr body. Which of the following best explains this finding?

(A) Laboratory error
(B) The patient is a male
(C) Classic XO pattern
(D) Turner's mosaic pattern
(E) Klinefelter's syndrome

41. Normal levels of C-reactive protein (CRP) are most often observed in

(A) acute viral illness
(B) pneumococcal pneumonia
(C) active rheumatoid arthritis
(D) active pulmonary tuberculosis
(E) acute myocardial infarction

42. The most specific of the commonly used tests for diagnosing active syphilis is the

(A) rapid plasma reagin (RPR) test
(B) *Treponema pallidum* immobilization (TPI) test
(C) fluorescent treponemal antibody-absorption (FTA-ABS) test
(D) Venereal Disease Research Laboratory (VDRL) test
(E) Kolmer test

43. Characteristic features of lepromatous leprosy include all the following EXCEPT

(A) nerve involvement
(B) numerous bacilli in histiocytes
(C) frequent polyclonal hypergammaglobulinemia
(D) association with erythema nodosum
(E) encroachment of infiltrate on basal epidermis

44. As visualized by the electron microscope, all the following are cell organelles EXCEPT

(A) lysosomes
(B) the Golgi complex
(C) the endoplasmic reticulum
(D) desmosomes
(E) microbodies

45. Spirochetal infections include all the following EXCEPT

(A) bejel
(B) yaws
(C) relapsing fever
(D) Weil's disease
(E) lymphogranuloma venereum

46. An elevated IgG level in cerebro-spinal fluid and an abnormal band on agar gel electrophoresis of cerebrospinal fluid are findings consistent with the diagnosis of

(A) secondary stage of syphilis
(B) muscular dystrophy
(C) tumor involvement of the spinal cord
(D) meningeal involvement by leukemia
(E) multiple sclerosis

47. Which of the following conditions is most likely to be associated with a negative result on routine pregnancy tests?

(A) Ectopic pregnancy
(B) Hydatidiform mole
(C) Polyhydramnios
(D) Eclampsia
(E) Choriocarcinoma

48. The texture and resilience of a given tumor grossly (macroscopically) are largely influenced by which of the following?

(A) Presence or absence of connective tissue stroma
(B) Degree of malignancy
(C) Interface between normal tissue and tumor
(D) Type of epithelium present
(E) Relative blood supply

49. A 37-year-old woman who has a clinical picture of fever, splenomegaly, varying neurologic manifestations, and purplish ecchymoses of the skin is found to have a hemoglobin level of 10.0 g/dl, a mean corpuscular hemo-globin concentration (MCHC) of 48, peripheral blood polychromasia with stippled macrocytes, and spherocytes, with a blood urea nitrogen level of 68 mg/dl. The findings of coagulation studies and the patient's fibrin-degraded products are not overtly abnormal. Which of the following is most closely identified with these findings?

(A) Idiopathic thrombocytopenic purpura
(B) Thrombotic thrombocytopenic purpura
(C) Disseminated intravascular coagu-lopathy
(D) Submassive hepatic necrosis
(E) Waterhouse-Friderichsen syndrome

50. The "stat" laboratory sends the following electrolyte results to the ward concerning a new admission: Na^+, 142 mEq/L; K^+, 7.2 mEq/L; Cl^-, 101 mEq/L; and CO_2, 32 mEq/L. On the basis of these results, the physician should

(A) treat with sodium exchange resin
(B) institute peritoneal dialysis imme-diately
(C) inquire about a hemolyzed blood sample
(D) infuse insulin intravenously
(E) make a diagnosis of hyperkalemia

51. Parathyroid hormone, by its action on target organs, is known to cause all the following EXCEPT

(A) increased intestinal calcium absorption
(B) increased renal tubular reabsorption of calcium
(C) increased serum phosphate levels
(D) mobilization of calcium from bone
(E) decreased renal tubular reabsorption of phosphate

52. The enzyme activity curve labeled II, shown below, best represents the pattern for which of the following serum enzymes after an uncomplicated acute myocardial infarction?

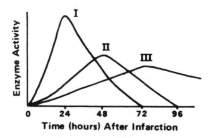

(A) Glutamic-oxaloacetic transaminase
(B) Creatine phosphokinase
(C) Lactic dehydrogenase
(D) Alkaline phosphatase
(E) 5′-Nucleotidase

53. A 65-year-old known diabetic man is admitted with fever, dehydration, and altered consciousness, with no perceptible odor of acetone on his breath. The serum Na^+ level is 146 mEq/L, the glucose level is 960 mg/dl, and the blood urea nitrogen level is 48 mg/dl. Calculate the serum osmolality.

(A) 280 mOsm
(B) 310 mOsm
(C) 318 mOsm
(D) 356 mOsm
(E) Insufficient data

54. Beriberi is associated with all the following conditions EXCEPT

(A) alcoholism
(B) thiamine deficiency
(C) diets of raw fish
(D) diets of polished rice
(E) diets low in fruit content

55. Which of the following assays is the most reliable and cost-effective screening method in separating Cushing's syndrome from conditions with similar features, such as obesity?

(A) Urinary 17-ketosteroids
(B) Urinary 17-ketogenic steroids
(C) Urinary 17-hydroxysteroids
(D) Urinary free cortisol
(E) Plasma cortisol

56. A lower-than-normal level of serum amylase is most typical of patients who have

(A) diabetes mellitus
(B) mumps
(C) renal insufficiency
(D) a ruptured ectopic pregnancy
(E) administration of morphine

57. What is the creatinine clearance of a person who passes 361 mg of creatinine in a 24-hour urine sample of 770 ml and whose plasma creatinine is 2.0 mg/100 ml?

(A) 12.5 ml/min
(B) 25.0 ml/min
(C) 50.0 ml/min
(D) 75.0 ml/min
(E) 100.0 ml/min

58. Hyperuricemia often occurs secondary to all the following disorders EXCEPT

(A) myeloproliferative disorders
(B) carcinoma
(C) chondrocalcinosis (pseudogout)
(D) starvation
(E) chronic renal disease

59. A 20-year-old student has an upper respiratory infection with severe sore throat and pain on swallowing. Her dormitory roommates make a diagnosis of infectious mononucleosis, thus saving her a trip to Student Health. Six weeks later, she develops a low-grade fever and back pain. A urinalysis finding of red blood cell casts

(A) reflects glomerular damage
(B) is insignificant if few casts are present
(C) is probably due to a menstrual "contaminant"
(D) suggests the presence of hemorrhagic cystitis
(E) is present in any instance of hematuria

60. While many factors come into play in a tumor's behavior, which of the following can be expected to influence the biology of a given tumor the *most*?

(A) Lack of a peripheral capsule
(B) Histologic differentiation
(C) Presence of inflammation
(D) Size of the tumor
(E) Nuclear cytoplasmic ratio

61. Elevated levels of alkaline phosphatase are typical findings in each of the following conditions EXCEPT

(A) cirrhosis
(B) obstructive jaundice
(C) hepatitis
(D) polycythemia vera
(E) myocardial infarction

62. An adult patient suffers from recurrent bleeding from the gums, intermittent GI bleeding, and excessive bleeding from minor trauma to the skin. A prolonged bleeding time is discovered. Which of the following levels or activities should be assessed to complete the diagnosis?

(A) Prothrombin time
(B) Plasma fibrinogen
(C) Factor VIII:R
(D) Factor VIII:C
(E) Factor VIII:Ag

63. The table below shows the normal serum values for the five isoenzymes of lactic dehydrogenase (LDH) and the values obtained for one patient. The diagnosis most compatible with the patient's values is

Isoenzyme	Normal % activity	Patient's % activity
LDH_1	20-35	18
LDH_2	30-40	24
LDH_3	20-30	13
LDH_4	5-15	26
LDH_5	1-15	19

(A) acute hepatitis
(B) pernicious anemia
(C) pulmonary infarct
(D) myocardial infarct
(E) cerebrovascular accident

64. An African boy with a rapidly expanding mass in the region of the jaw and cheek is thought to have Burkitt's lymphoma. These cells are growing rapidly because of

(A) their permanent nature
(B) shortening of the cell cycle
(C) nonsequencing of the EBV genome
(D) fewer G_0 cells entering the cycle
(E) delayed progression from G_2 to mitosis

65. Environmental and industrial pollutants are becoming increasingly relevant in human oncogenesis. Which of the following combinations is most closely allied with human neoplasia?

(A) Asbestos, silica, arsenicals
(B) Diethylstilbestrol, radioactive dusts, cyanide
(C) Aflatoxin, beryllium vapor, benzidine
(D) Polyvinyl chloride, nickel, chromium
(E) Carbon tetrachloride, lead, chloroform

66. Which of the following is physiologically the most active thyroid hormone?

(A) Thyroglobulin
(B) Monoiodotyrosine (MIT)
(C) Diiodotyrosine (DIT)
(D) Triiodothyronine (T_3)
(E) Thyroxine (T_4)

67. A diagnosis of adrenogenital syndrome with demonstrable adrenal hyperplasia is consistent with

(A) generalized calcium oxalate deposition similar to that occurring in oxalosis
(B) accumulation of glycolipids in tissues
(C) salt loss simulating Addison's disease
(D) symptoms similar to those occurring in phenylketonuria
(E) severe acidosis

68. In Tay-Sachs disease, the ganglioside that accumulates specific to the
disease lacks

(A) sphingosine
(B) the terminal galactose unit
(C) the fatty acid moiety
(D) a hexosamine moiety
(E) the entire carbohydrate moiety

69. A 21-year-old woman with recurrent painful crises in the extremities
and an inability to sweat is found to
have multiple vascular lesions of the
abdomen and thigh and corneal opacity
on slit-lamp examination. Which of the
following conditions is suggested by
these findings?

(A) Fabry's disease
(B) Fanconi syndrome
(C) Tay-Sachs disease
(D) Hand-Schüller-Christian disease
(E) Gaucher's disease

70. A chromosomal aberration that results in a disturbance in the normal
gene balance is termed

(A) nondisjunction
(B) euploidy
(C) aneuploidy
(D) breakage
(E) variance

71. The major underlying defect in
classical renal tubular acidosis (caused
by gradient defect) appears to be

(A) an excessive back-diffusion of secreted hydrogen ions from tubular
urine to blood
(B) an impairment of ammonia excretion
(C) a leakage of bicarbonate ions out
of the proximal tubule
(D) a deficiency in the total hydrogen
ion secretory capacity
(E) an impairment in the reclamation
of filtered bicarbonate ions

72. Lobar pneumonia is caused predominantly by

(A) *Klebsiella pneumoniae*
(B) *Staphylococcus pyogenes*
(C) *Hemophilus influenzae*
(D) *Streptococcus pneumoniae*
(E) *Legionella pneumophila*

73. Relatively nonpathogenic pneumo-
cocci typically exhibit

(A) R (rough) genotypes
(B) positive quellung reactions
(C) alpha-hemolysis when grown on
blood agar
(D) bile-solubility when grown in de-
oxycholate media
(E) positive reactions on exposure to
type 3 antisera

74. Characteristically, B lymphocytes do all the following EXCEPT

(A) constitute 10 to 15 percent of peripheral blood lymphocytes
(B) occur in lymphoid follicles and the superficial cortex of lymph nodes
(C) express surface immunoglobulins IgM and IgD
(D) express cluster differentiation antigen CD8
(E) possess complement component (C3) receptors

75. Which of the following organisms produces signs and symptoms that mimic acute appendicitis?

(A) Enteropathic *Escherichia coli*
(B) *Enterobius vermicularis*
(C) *Trichomonas hominis*
(D) *Yersinia enterocolitica*
(E) *Bacillus anthracis*

76. An adult migrant farm worker in the San Joaquin Valley of California has been hospitalized for 2 weeks on the medical service with progressing lassitude, fever of unknown origin, and skin nodules on the lower extremities. A biopsy of one of the deep dermal nodules shown in the photomicrograph below reveals the presence of

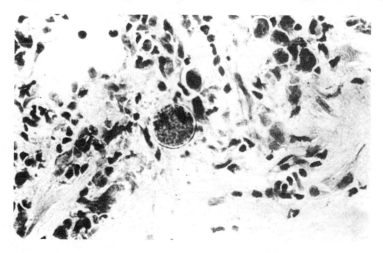

(A) Russell bodies
(B) malignant lymphoma
(C) coccidioides spherule
(D) lymphomatoid granulomatosis
(E) erythema nodosum

77. Delayed-type hypersensitivity reactions of the tuberculin skin test type

(A) appear within 1 or 2 hours
(B) require an intact T-lymphocyte population
(C) show dermal infiltrates of granulocytes
(D) are associated uniquely with small antigens
(E) do not require previous exposure to the antigen

78. Large amounts of antigen are required to produce

(A) serum sickness
(B) an Arthus reaction
(C) generalized anaphylaxis
(D) cutaneous anaphylaxis
(E) atopic responses

79. Unusual characteristics of mycobacteria, such as resistance to toxic agents, environmental viability, and unusual stain reactions, can be attributed to their

(A) acid fastness
(B) aerobic requirements
(C) high lipid content
(D) peptidoglycan content
(E) plasma membrane

80. Togaviruses cause all the following disorders EXCEPT

(A) epidemic keratoconjunctivitis
(B) dengue
(C) eastern encephalitis
(D) yellow fever
(E) St. Louis encephalitis

81. All the following statements about *Mycobacterium tuberculosis* are true EXCEPT

(A) it has a long doubling time
(B) its cell wall contains large amounts of lipid
(C) it frequently infects silica miners
(D) it is prone to drug-resistant mutation
(E) it is a facultative anaerobe

82. Which of the following organisms is highly pathogenic in humans, grows as an encapsulated yeast both in culture and in infected tissues, and often produces a chronic, exudative meningitis?

(A) *Aspergillus fumigatus*
(B) *Histoplasma capsulatum*
(C) *Coccidioides immitis*
(D) *Cryptococcus neoformans*
(E) *Blastomyces dermatitidis*

83. The organism *Mycoplasma pneumoniae* exhibits all the following characteristics EXCEPT which one?

(A) It is enclosed by a membrane, but lacks cell walls
(B) It causes 50 percent of pneumonias in college students
(C) It is often accompanied by the presence of cold agglutinins in serum
(D) It is beyond resolution of light microscopy
(E) It causes granuloma formation

84. All the following diseases are associated with herpesviruses EXCEPT

(A) shingles
(B) chickenpox (varicella)
(C) influenza
(D) cytomegalic inclusion disease
(E) mononucleosis

85. A woman taking oral contraceptives during the reproductive years increases, even if only minimally, her risk of developing all the following EXCEPT

(A) pulmonary infarction
(B) myocardial infarction
(C) vaginal adenosis
(D) venous thrombus
(E) liver cell adenoma

86. Alcohol may be the most significant cause of public health problems in the United States. All the following entities are correlated with alcohol abuse EXCEPT

(A) subdural hematoma
(B) esophageal carcinoma
(C) elevated creatine phosphokinase
(D) primary biliary cirrhosis
(E) portal vein thrombosis

87. All the following statements about *Listeria monocytogenes* are true EXCEPT that it

(A) causes neonatal and adult meningitis
(B) causes food-borne outbreaks
(C) causes frequent epithelioid granulomas
(D) is an opportunistic agent in the immunosuppressed or pregnant
(E) is a gram-positive intracellular bacillus

88. Current knowledge concerning AIDS (acquired immunodeficiency syndrome) includes all the following EXCEPT

(A) the causative agent is HIV
(B) the causative agent belongs to the retrovirus group
(C) T lymphocytes of the helper/inducer subset are infected
(D) cytotoxic/suppressor T cells are markedly increased
(E) lymphoid interstitial pneumonitis is seen in pediatric AIDS

DIRECTIONS: Each question below contains four suggested responses of which **one or more** is correct. Select

A	if	**1, 2, and 3**	are correct
B	if	**1 and 3**	are correct
C	if	**2 and 4**	are correct
D	if	**4**	is correct
E	if	**1, 2, 3, and 4**	are correct

89. A 54-year-old woman with a 30 pack-year history of cigarette smoking underwent a bronchial biopsy after a central mass was seen on x-ray. The photomicrograph below shows the biopsy result. This disorder is demonstrated in which of the following paraneoplastic syndromes?

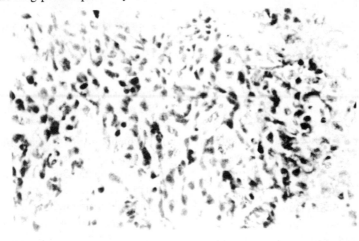

(1) Cushing's syndrome
(2) Hyponatremia
(3) Carcinoid syndrome
(4) Hypercalcemia

90. A significant deficiency in vitamin D might be expected to lead to

(1) osteomalacia
(2) relative excess of osteoid tissue
(3) decreased absorption of calcium
(4) decreased production of bone matrix

91. Infectious diseases associated with a granulomatous response include

(1) tuberculosis
(2) coccidioidomycosis
(3) schistosomiasis
(4) sarcoidosis

92. True statements regarding celiac disease include that

(1) there is an increased frequency of HLA-B8 and HLA-Dw3 antigens
(2) mucosal changes on immunoperoxidase staining and electron microscopy are pathognomonic
(3) long-standing disease is associated with an increased incidence of gastrointestinal malignancy
(4) jejunal biopsy shows villous atrophy and decreased mitotic activity in crypts

93. Epstein-Barr virus (EBV) infections can be associated with neoplastic states. In infectious mononucleosis, control of the EBV infected cells is effected by which of the following factors?

(1) B cell membrane antigen
(2) Macrophage migration inhibitory factor
(3) Increase in T killer cells
(4) Lack of EBV replication

---

94. The photomicrograph below shows a labeling phenomenon of dark cytoplasmic granules within select cells. This staining technique

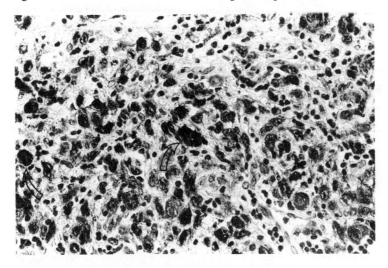

(1) relies on neutral polysaccharides for a positive reaction
(2) relies on antigen-antibody binding
(3) stains neutral and acid mucopolysaccharides
(4) may be used to identify tumor cell markers

SUMMARY OF DIRECTIONS

A	B	C	D	E
1, 2, 3 only	1, 3 only	2, 4 only	4 only	All are correct

95. True statements about endometrial adenocarcinoma include which of the following?

(1) It is more common than invasive squamous cervical cancer
(2) It causes fewer deaths than invasive cervical cancer
(3) The peak incidence is at age 55 to 65 years
(4) Abnormal glucose tolerance is a risk factor

96. Fat necrosis is a characteristic histologic change associated with

(1) acute pancreatitis
(2) hyperlipidemia
(3) traumatized breast tissue
(4) hibernomas

97. Secondary gout may be seen in association with

(1) polycythemia
(2) psoriasis
(3) hemolytic anemias
(4) myeloproliferative diseases

98. Atherosclerosis, the most prevalent form of arterial disease in humans, is first manifested by an innocuous fatty streaking of the intima and is characterized by

(1) formation of essential lesions in the intima
(2) disintegration of the internal elastic lamina in advanced lesions
(3) relatively numerous lesions in larger arteries and fewer in smaller arteries
(4) plaque formations that cause little reduction in the luminal size of large arteries

99. Glycogen storage diseases include which of the following?

(1) Von Gierke's disease
(2) Pompe's disease
(3) McArdle's disease
(4) Tay-Sachs disease

100. Characteristics of granular cell tumors commonly include

(1) location in the tongue
(2) PAS-positive, diastase-resistant granules
(3) association with pseudoepitheliomatous hyperplasia
(4) origin from myoblastic cells

101. Pyridoxine (vitamin B_6) deficiency is known to be associated with

(1) synthesis of neurotransmitters
(2) mental retardation
(3) peripheral neuropathies
(4) degeneration of ganglion cells

102. True statements regarding hemo-chromatosis include which of the following?

(1) It characteristically causes a macronodular pigment cirrhosis
(2) It is complicated by carcinoma of the liver in 15 to 30 percent of cases with cirrhosis
(3) It causes diabetes with severity directly related to the degree of pancreatic iron deposition
(4) It can be diagnosed by liver biopsy showing raised amounts of hemosiderin

103. As a result of active world travel, parasitic infestations are far from being considered exotic diseases in the United States today. A pulmonary phase is part of the development of which of the following helminths?

(1) *Necator americanus*
(2) *Strongyloides stercoralis*
(3) *Ascaris lumbricoides*
(4) *Wuchereria bancrofti*

---

104. Which of the following functions can be attributed to the cell depicted in the electron photomicrograph below?

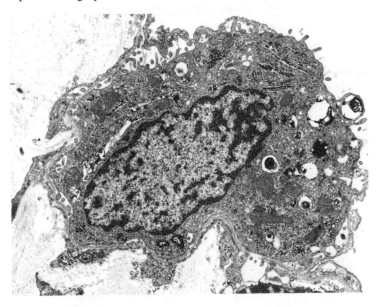

(1) Production of thromboplastin
(2) Degranulation in type I reactions
(3) Production of interleukin I
(4) Factor VIII-vWF synthesis

SUMMARY OF DIRECTIONS				
A	B	C	D	E
1, 2, 3 only	1, 3 only	2, 4 only	4 only	All are correct

105. Taking patient discomfort and expense into account, bone marrow aspiration and trephine examination are indicated to document

(1) metastatic carcinoma
(2) iron deficiency anemia
(3) sideroblastic anemia
(4) osteoporosis

106. An increased incidence of neoplasia has been observed in

(1) primary (genetic) immunodeficient states
(2) immunosuppressed recipients of transplants
(3) acquired immunodeficiency syndrome (AIDS)
(4) therapy with radiation and radiomimetic drugs

107. Organisms that can cause summertime infections around coastal areas of the United States and are characterized microscopically by a curved bacillus include

(1) *Mycobacterium avium*
(2) *Mycobacterium bovis*
(3) *Mycobacterium marinum*
(4) *Vibrio cholerae*

108. Leukotrienes differ from prostaglandins in the mediation of inflammation by their more potent actions of

(1) chemotaxis
(2) vasoconstriction
(3) bronchoconstriction
(4) edema formation

DIRECTIONS: Each group of questions below consists of lettered headings followed by a set of numbered items. For each numbered item select the **one** lettered heading with which it is **most** closely associated. Each lettered heading may be used **once, more than once, or not at all.**

Questions 109-111

Tumor markers and paraneoplastic syndromes are helpful in diagnosis, monitoring therapy, and prognosis of specific types of tumors. For each tumor listed below, select the marker or syndrome most likely to assist in diagnosis.

(A) Desmin
(B) Acanthosis nigricans
(C) Alpha-fetoprotein
(D) Polycythemia
(E) Acid phosphatase

109. Gastric carcinoma

110. Renal cell carcinoma

111. Prostatic carcinoma

Questions 112-115

Match the following characteristics and diseases.

(A) Tick-borne disease
(B) Granulomatous inflammation
(C) Leonine facies
(D) Mosquito-borne disease
(E) Endotoxins in cell walls

112. Histoplasmosis

113. Lepromatous leprosy

114. Rocky Mountain spotted fever

115. Yellow fever

Questions 116-119

For each disease causative of blindness, select the characteristic with which it is most likely to be associated.

(A) Silver-wire arterioles
(B) Variable modes of inheritance
(C) Microaneurysms
(D) Bitot's spots
(E) Pannus formation

116. Diabetic retinopathy

117. Keratomalacia

118. Trachoma

119. Retinitis pigmentosa

Questions 120-123

Match each disorder or description with the immunoglobulin with which it is most likely to be associated.

(A) IgA
(B) IgD
(C) IgE
(D) IgM
(E) IgG

120. Anaphylaxis

121. The major circulating immunoglobulin

122. Berger's disease

123. Waldenström's macroglobulinemia

General Pathology
Answers

1. The answer is A. *(Robbins, ed 4. pp 31-33.)* In uterine growth during pregnancy, both cell proliferation involving the endometrial glands and muscle enlargement of the uterine wall occur. These processes offer models of both hyperplasia and hypertrophy. When both are present, DNA synthesis is markedly accelerated. Hyperplasia is an increase in the number of cells, whereas hypertrophy is an increase in cell size, as in cardiac muscle hypertrophy in response to volume overload or peripheral vascular hypertension. Breast tissue enlargement resulting from hormonal influences is due solely to an increase in cell numbers.

2. The answer is C. *(Robbins, ed 4. pp 78-80, 138-139.)* Type I collagen is found in skin, tendon, bone, dentin, and fascia; type II collagen is found only in cartilage; type III collagen (reticulin) appears in skin, blood vessels, uterus, and embryonic dermis. Type IV collagen, a component of basement laminae of epithelial and endothelial cells, does not have the typical 67-nm banding of types I, II, and III. Synthesis of collagen includes lysine oxidation, resulting in alpha-chain cross-linkages with structural stability of collagen. Decreased formation of cross-linkages in collagen and elastin occurs in Marfan's syndrome, an autosomal dominant disorder of connective tissues, with skeletal abnormalities including arachnodactyly, lens subluxation, and cystic medionecrosis of aorta with aneurysm and sometimes rupture.

3. The answer is B. *(Robbins, ed 4. pp 4-9.)* Injury to the cell membrane, the loss of cell ATP, and the influx of Ca^{2+} into the mitochondria are thought to be the most critical of multiple cellular events after experimental ischemia in animals. A major detriment following reduction of cell oxygen tension is the cessation or reduction in ATP because of falling oxidative phosphorylation; this occurs early in hypoxia. While increasing anaerobic glycolysis subsequently occurs, the pivotal step is loss of the energy-producing ATP, which leads to cell Na^+ accumulation, K^+ efflux, and Ca^{2+} influx, by reduced effectiveness of the active transport Na^+ pump. Cells greatly enlarge as a consequence of isoosmotic water accumulation. These changes are still reversible if oxygen tension is restored. Continuing hypoxia results in mitochondrial damage (vacuole formation), which is irreversible. Cell death will occur when lysosomes break down and release proteases, RNA and DNAases, and cathepsins. Central nervous system cells are most susceptible to ischemia (5 minutes or less), while liver and kidney cells survive up to 2 hours with epidermal cells tolerating several hours of hypoxia.

4. The answer is E. *(Robbins, ed 4. pp 45-46.)* Leukocyte function antigen-1 (LFA-1) is one of the group of adhesive molecules on leukocytes. Other members of this group, all glycoproteins and all having identical β chains, are MO-1 and P-150. A genetic deficiency of these β-chain adhesive proteins on leukocytes (leukocyte adhesion deficiency) results in impaired leukocyte adhesion and recurrent bacterial infections. Endothelial leukocyte adhesion molecule (ELAM-1) is one of the adhesive surface proteins on endothelial cells. Complement fragments (C5a) and leukotriene B4 are mediators that stimulate an increase in adhesive molecules on *leukocytes*. Conversely, interleukin-1 (IL-1) stimulates leukocytic adhesion by action on adhesive surface proteins on *endothelial* cells. Tumor necrosis factor (TNF) stimulates adhesive molecules on *both* leukocytes and endothelial cells.

5. The answer is C. *(Robbins, ed 4. pp 58-60, 70-71, 168-169, 183.)* Two of the major systemic effects of inflammation (acute-phase reactions) are fever and leukocytosis. Both of these reactions are largely under the control of the cytokines IL-1 or α-TNF (cachectin) or both. These two cytokines have many similar functions, including induction of fever, release of ACTH, leukocytosis, and other systemic acute-phase responses. IL-1 initiates fever by inducing synthesis of prostaglandin E_2 (PGE_2) in the anterior hypothalamus, followed by transmission via the posterior hypothalamus, vasomotor center, and sympathetic nerves to cause skin vasoconstriction. Leukocytosis occurs initially because of rapid release of cells from the postmitotic reserve pool of the bone marrow, caused by IL-1 and α-TNF and associated with a "shift to the left" of immature cells. β-TNF, another cytokine, has no major role in acute-phase reactions. It takes part in T-cell cytotoxicity and its release may injure cell membranes directly in T-cell-mediated lysis.

6. The answer is B. *(Robbins, ed 4. pp 51-52.)* The enzymatic defect that exists in chronic granulomatous disease of childhood does not impair chemotaxis or the cell's ability to engulf bacteria, but rather involves a failure to produce hydrogen peroxide after engulfment. Chemotactic defects resulting in inhibition of the capacity of leukocytes to infiltrate an area of infection or injury may be due to intracellular defects, as found in Chédiak-Higashi syndrome, in other genetic defects, and in diabetes mellitus. Chronic renal failure and other liver disease may be associated with factors in the circulation that impair chemotaxis. Whether newborn infants are full-term or immature, neonatal leukocytes have a temporary chemotactic defect that is corrected with increasing age.

7. The answer is C. *(Takahashi, ed 2. pp 305-306.)* In the cluster of cells shown, marked variation in cell size, nuclear hyperchromatism, and prominent nuclear membranes can be seen and are diagnostic characteristics of malignancy. The tendency of cells to cluster and overlap, the prominent nucleoli, and the vacuolated cytoplasm are signs that strongly support a diagnosis of adenocarcinoma rather than oat cell carcinoma.

8.   The answer is C. *(Robbins, ed 4. pp 29-30, 51-52.)* Cytoskeletal filament proteins compose the framework of cells involved in cell functions, such as pinocytosis, structural stability, contractility, organelle movement, and cell motility. The cytoskeleton is seen ultrastructurally as microtubules (25 nm diameter) of tubulin protein; intermediate filaments (8 to 10 nm) of keratins, desmin, vimentin, glial and neurofilaments; thin filaments of actin (6 to 8 nm); and thick filaments (15 nm) of myosin. Every cell has tubulin and actin, while most have some myosin. Epithelial cells have any of the many types of cytokeratins, with a few having the mesenchymal filament vimentin. Muscle cells and fibroblasts have desmin. Glial cells and neurons contain glial and neurofilament protein, respectively. Phagocytosis is impaired in the Chédiak-Higashi syndrome because of a defect in the polymerization of microtubules. Alcoholic "hyaline" (Mallory's bodies) in alcoholic liver disease appears to be composed of prekeratins. Red cells have a membrane skeleton made up of spectrin, ankyrin, actin, and protein 4.1. In hereditary spherocytosis a genetic defect is responsible for abnormal spectrin that is unable to bind protein 4.1 required for the stability of the red cell membrane.

9.   The answer is D. *(Robbins, ed 4. pp 114-119.)* Septic shock is caused by the gram-negative, endotoxin-producing aerobic rods mentioned in the question. It results from pooling of blood in the peripheral circulation. A common cause of sepsis in burn wounds is *Pseudomonas aeruginosa*. The major target in severe shock is the kidneys, which suffer acute ischemic tubular necrosis, affecting proximal and distal nephrons in septic shock. Gram-negative endotoxic shock has a 70 percent mortality.

10.   The answer is D. *(Anderson, ed 9. pp 2154-2156. Henry, ed 17. p 474.)* In a patient who is suspected of having meningitis, microscopic examination of cerebrospinal fluid is of immediate importance. In the photomicrograph shown, all the cells are polymorphonuclear leukocytes and bacteria are visible in the cytoplasm. Neutrophils may be present in viral or tuberculous meningitis, but lymphocytes are more common. Demonstration of bacteria by Gram stain of the cerebrospinal fluid is the most valuable aid in establishing a diagnosis of early bacterial meningitis and is possible in more than 90 percent of cases.

11.   The answer is E. *(Robbins, ed 4. pp 52-60.)* Lysosomes contain many substances involved in inflammation including alkaline and acid phosphatase, collagenases, lysozymes, lactoferrin, myeloperoxidase, cationic proteins, and acid proteases. Of these, the neutral proteases (elastase, collagenase, cathepsin G) function in stages of inflammatory confinement and wound healing by degrading tissue matrix like collagen, fibrin, cartilage, elastin, and basement membranes. The other mediators cascade as follows: complement cascade starts classically by an antigen-antibody complex or alternately by nonimmunologic stimuli. C5a leads to chemotaxis while the complement complex C5b-9 leads to cell lysis. The kinins are activated by Hageman factor (XIIA), via prekallikrein, into bradykinin. The fibrinopeptides of the clotting system can also be activated by Hageman factor or by extrinsic tissue thromboplastin to result in a polymerized fibrin clot. The important cascades of arachidonic acid metabolites (cyclooxygenase, lipoxygenase), leading to functioning vasodilators (prostaglandins) and membrane permeability factors (leukotrienes), are the most complex of all, beginning with the actions of phospholipase.

12. The answer is C. *(Robbins, ed 3. pp 818-821.)* Squamous cell (epidermoid) carcinoma is the most common oral malignancy (97 percent). Half of the cases arise in the tongue, with the lower lip and the floor of the mouth the next most frequent sites. This carcinoma occurs predominantly in men of age 40 and over; heavy tobacco and alcohol use are risk factors. It may form a red or white lesion and should be differentiated from lichen planus, keratoacanthoma, and necrotizing sialometaplasia (difficult!). Metastases may be bilateral to neck lymph nodes, as in laryngeal squamous cancer.

13. The answer is D. *(Anderson, ed 9. pp 438-439.)* *Giardia lamblia*, a flagellate protozoan, is the most common cause of outbreaks of waterborne diarrheal disease in the U.S. and is seen frequently in Rocky Mountain areas. Ingestion of cysts from contaminated water results in trophozoites in duodenum and jejunum. Identification of the trophozoite stage is done by duodenal aspiration or small-bowel biopsy and of the cyst stage (intermittent) by examination of stool. The trophozoite may appear as a pear-shaped, binucleate organism ("two eyes"). Giardiasis may cause malabsorption but is often asymptomatic. Duodenal aspiration, immunofluorescence, and ELISA testing for *Giardia* antigens are diagnostic and therapy with metronidazole or quinacrine is effective. Lymph nodes often contain numerous parasites in trypanosomiasis and leishmaniasis. *Triatoma* is the vector of Chagas' disease (American trypanosomiasis). *Trichomonas vaginalis* is identified in cervicovaginal smears.

14. The answer is C. *(Robbins, ed 4. pp 1374-1375.)* Liposarcomas are the most common soft tissue sarcoma of adults, arise deeply in thigh or retroperitoneum, and are liable to metastasize by embolization in blood vessels (nonmyxoid types). Histology is varied: well-differentiated, myxoid, round cell, or pleomorphic— depending on tumor type. Myxoid liposarcoma is the most common variant. The pleomorphic type is undifferentiated and easily confused with other poorly differentiated mesenchymal sarcomas. The clinical picture is also varied. Well-differentiated and myxoid types are locally invasive and recurrent, if they are not completely excised, but they are rarely metastatic. Round-cell and pleomorphic types are often aggressive with widespread metastases, local recurrence, and poor 5-year survival.

15. The answer is D. *(Robbins, ed 4. pp 61-63.)* There is evidence that most, if not all, macrophages originate from a committed bone marrow stem cell, which differentiates into a monoblast and then a promonocyte, which in turn matures into a monocyte in the circulating peripheral blood. When called upon, the circulating monocyte can enter into any organ or tissue bed as a tissue macrophage (previously called a histiocyte). Examples of tissue macrophages are Kupffer cells (liver), alveolar macrophages (lung), osteoclasts (bone), Langerhans cells (skin), microglial cells (central nervous system), and possibly the dendritic immunocytes of the dermis, spleen, and lymph nodes. The entire system, including the peripheral blood monocytes, constitutes the mononuclear phagocyte system.

16. The answer is B. *(Anderson, ed 9. p 1474.)* The lymph-node section shown in the photomicrograph contains metastatic carcinoma cells and was probably excised from a patient who has carcinoma. The tumor cells are clustered in small nests within the node and are separated by stromal tissue. The cellular clustering is characteristic of carcinomas that have metastasized to lymph nodes.

17. The answer is A. *(Robbins, ed 4. pp 146-148.)* Sphingomyelin, a lipid composed of phosphocholine and a ceramide, characteristically is found in abnormally high concentrations throughout the body tissues of patients who have any one of the forms of Niemann-Pick disease. Division of this disease into five categories is generally accepted; type A, the acute neuronopathic form, is the one that has the highest incidence. The lack of sphingomyelinase in type A is the metabolic defect that prevents the hydrolytic cleavage of sphingomyelin, which then accumulates in the brain. Patients who have the type A form usually show hepatosplenomegaly at 6 months of age, progressively lose motor functions and mental capabilities, and die during the third year of life.

18. The answer is B. *(Robbins, ed 4. pp 745-747.)* The Hand-Schüller-Christian (HSC) disease is a complex of three syndromes affecting the reticuloendothelial system: Letterer-Siwe syndrome, Hand-Schüller-Christian syndrome, and eosinophilic granuloma. An unknown pathogenesis and an abnormal production of histiocytes are characteristics common to all three syndromes and provide the basis for the designation of HSC disease as *histiocytosis X* (the alternate term is *Langerhans cell granulomatosis,* since the cells have the Birbeck granules ultrastructurally, as do Langerhans cells).

19. The answer is E. *(Robbins, ed 4. pp 1377-1378.)* Fibrosarcomas are most frequent in the retroperitoneum, followed by the superficial or deep tissues of the extremities. They form one of the less common tumors of soft tissue since many previously diagnosed as fibrosarcoma have been reclassified as malignant fibrous histiocytoma or aggressive fibromatosis (desmoid). Slowly growing, well-differentiated fibrosarcomas may be difficult to differentiate from "cellular fibromas." Hypoglycemia may be associated with fibrosarcoma.

20. The answer is A. *(Anderson, ed 9. p 874.)* The findings of small, firm testes, eunuchoidism, gynecomastia, and mental retardation constitute the classic manifestations of Klinefelter's syndrome, a type of hypogonadism. The seminiferous tubules may be sclerosed and hyalinized. Urinary levels of gonadotropin are usually elevated; the elevation is thought to result from the absence of controlling testicular hormones, not from pituitary dysfunction.

21. The answer is B. *(Robbins, ed 4. pp 127, 136.)* Mendel's laws deal with single-gene mutations that may be inherited or acquired de novo, with expression of the abnormality highly variable. In autosomal dominance inheritances, if a mutant gene is unexpressed, this is called *reduced penetrance* and it may vary by a percentage that reflects the degree of expression. *Variable expressivity* refers to expression of the trait in all who harbor the mutant gene, but with different expressions of the abnormality. *Nondisjunction* refers to a failure of disjoining of a homologous pair of chromosomes during meiosis (may result in aneuploidy). *Codominance* refers to the full expression of both alleles of a gene pair. *Genetic heterogeneity* applies to multiple-loci mutations (each in a different location, reflecting multiple different mutations), which can result in the same or similar expressed abnormality.

22. The answer is A. *(Robbins, ed 4. pp 51-52, 223.)* The classic form of chronic granulomatous disease usually afflicts boys and causes their death before they reach the age of 10 years. Key findings in chronic granulomatous disease include lymphadenitis, hepatosplenomegaly, eczematoid dermatitis, pulmonary infiltrates that are associated with hypergammaglobulinemia, and defective ability of neutrophils to kill bacteria. The last finding is thought to be caused by a delay in the release of neutrophilic lysosomal enzymes responsible for intracellular bactericidal action. Although defective neutrophilic bactericidal action also is associated with the Chédiak-Higashi syndrome, this syndrome is distinguished by photophobia and oculocutaneous albinism. Thrombocytopenia is a feature of Wiskott-Aldrich syndrome.

23. The answer is D. *(Robbins, ed 4. pp 267, 274.)* Mutations are alterations in the genetic code. The incidence of these alterations normally increases with age and is especially high in certain autosomal recessive disorders—e.g., Fanconi's anemia, ataxia telangiectasia, and Bloom's syndrome ("chromosome-breakage syndromes"). Persons with such disorders are highly susceptible to mutations due to such environmental influences as sunlight, ionizing radiation, drugs, viruses, and possibly elements in the diet (e.g., nitrite additives). It is thought that one mechanism operative in alterations in the genetic code is the binding of mutagenic substances directly to DNA guanine.

24. The answer is C. *(Robbins, ed 4. pp 29, 945-946.)* Hyaline inclusions, as shown in the illustration, may appear in liver cells injured by chronic alcoholism and have been shown by ultrastructure studies to result from the close packing of fibrils. The appearance of these inclusions is not a morphologic expression of cell injury. Alcoholic hyaline inclusions (Mallory's bodies) are nonspecific and occur in

Wilson's disease, Indian childhood cirrhosis, bypass operations for morbid obesity, and alcoholic hepatitis. They react with antibodies to cytokeratins, which suggests they are related to the intermediate filament keratin.

25. The answer is D. *(Robbins, ed 4. pp 177, 224-226, 296-297, 955-956.)* Newly discovered membrane surface antigens on the surfaces of neoplastic cells have stimulated interest and research. These tumor-associated antigens are largely glycoproteins (proteoglycans, chondroitins, heparin) that are at least anchored in the bilipid cell membrane with polypeptide chains emerging "into space" on the surface. Monoclonal antibodies can be raised against certain epitopes on the external portions of these surface antigens. Also the host may mount specific immunoglobulins against these sites. These antigens are membrane-associated, induce transplantation immunity, and are distinct from histocompatibility antigens; they are called tumor-specific transplantation antigens (TSTA) or tumor-associated rejection antigens (TARA). TSTA are found on tumor cells that were transformed by viral oncogenes. TSTA resemble differentiation antigens in normal cells of some animal strains. Most TSTA are related to carcinogens or oncogenes and are usually absent in spontaneous tumors. ADCC is antibody-dependent cell-mediated cytotoxicity; A1AT is alpha-1-antitrypsin. HIV is the designation of the AIDS retrovirus, while ARC is the AIDS-related complex.

26. The answer is E. *(Robbins, ed 4. p 259.)* Generally tumor cells, by virtue of their transformation, exhibit ultrastructural alterations as visualized by electron microscopy as well as physiologic changes. Membrane projections (microvilli, filopodia, pseudopodia) may become blunted, or lost altogether. Neoplastic transformation may be associated with formation of projections in some cells, but the loss of attenuation of surface projections is more characteristic of neoplastic cells. Cytoskeletal microfilaments and tubules become disorganized, while intermediate filaments (keratins, desmin, vimentin) may increase. In addition to formation of membrane-associated glycoproteins (tumor antigens), there is increased "shedding" and loss of surface antigens. Fibronectin, for instance, is lost from tumor cell surfaces and may be measured in the patient's plasma as cold-insoluble globulin. Surface glycolipids (many are receptor sites) are diminished or lost in some neoplastic cells, theoretically enabling tumor cells to escape the growth inhibitory effects of chalones. Plant lectins can agglutinate cells because their property of divalency cross-links sugars on neighboring cells. This lectin agglutinability is increased in many malignant cells. Fundamental to the biologic behavior of neoplastic cells is the increased demand for cell nutrients, which is aided by an observed increase in membrane transport in neoplastic cells.

27. The answer is A. *(Anderson, ed 9. p 492. Robbins, ed 4. pp 165-167.)* With the advent of monoclonal antibodies derived from hybridomas, it is now possible to identify cells of certain specificity. These antibodies recognize epitopes of antigens found on the cell surfaces that have been used to induce immunity within the mouse. Using an immunoperoxidase technique, the OKT (Leu series) identifies T cells. In addition specific markers will identify subsets of T cells: For example all peripheral blood T cells react with OKT1, OKT3, and OKT11 cluster designations CD5, CD3, and CD2; OKT4 (Leu-3) reacts with mature T cells; OKT4 or CD4 identifies helper T cells; and OKT8 (CD8) reacts with suppressor cells. The normal T helper/suppressor ratio in humans is about 2. These antibodies do not label cells other than those in the T-lymphocyte system. T cells as a group function in immune regulation and act in concert with B lymphocytes and macrophages. T helper cells aid the cellular immune response in reaction to antigens, while T suppressor cells help in turning the immune response off. EAC rosette cells refer to B lymphocytes that have surface receptors (C3b) that bind to sheep erythrocytes coated with IgM antibody and complement. B lymphocytes also express surface immunoglobulin.

28. The answer is B. *(Robbins, ed 4. pp 50-51, 167-168, 297, 299.)* The enzyme myeloperoxidase is found in high concentration in neutrophilic granulocytes and exerts strong antibacterial effects by combining with chloride and hydrogen peroxide. Natural killer (NK) cells are able to lyse certain tumor cells, virus-infected cells, fungi, and some normal cells without prior sensitization. It is now believed that most so-called killer (K) cells are really NK cells and K cells are now known as cytotoxic T cells. NK cells lyse target cells in two ways: through direct cytotoxicity by means of their NK receptors, and through antibody-dependent cytotoxicity (ADCC) by their Fc receptors for IgG. NK cells are sometimes called *large granular lymphocytes* (larger than small lymphocytes) and their granules contain lytic substances, but not myeloperoxidase. NK cells share some surface antigens with T cells and macrophages, but are considered distinct from these. Monoclonal antibodies reacting with NK cells include CD16. Following activation and increase in numbers by culture with interleukin-2, NK cells can kill many tumor cells, and these lymphokine-activated killer (LAK) cells are being evaluated in the immunotherapy of some cancers—leukemia, melanoma, renal cell carcinoma—currently treated with IL-2 and interferons.

29. The answer is D. *(Robbins, ed 4. pp 173-183.)* The type of reaction in the question is a type 2 hypersensitivity reaction that is mediated by antibodies reacting against antigens present on the surface of cells, in this case blood group antigens or irregular antigens present on the donor's red blood cells. Type 2 hypersensitivity reactions result from attachment of antibodies to changed cell surface antigens or to normal cell surface antigens. Complement-mediated cytotoxicity occurs when IgM or IgG binds to a cell surface antigen with complement activation and consequent cell membrane damage or lysis. Blood transfusion reactions and autoimmune hemolytic anemia are examples of this form. Systemic anaphylaxis is a type 1 hypersensitivity reaction in which mast cells or basophils that are bound to IgE antibodies are reexposed to an allergen, which leads to a release of vasoactive amines that causes edema and broncho- and vasoconstriction. Sudden death can occur. Systemic immune complex reactions are found in type 3 reactions and are due to circulating antibodies that form complexes upon reexposure to an antigen, such as foreign serum, which then activates complement followed by chemotaxis and aggregation of neutrophils leading to release of lysosomal enzymes and eventual necrosis of tissue and cells. Serum sickness and Arthus' reactions are examples of this. Delayed-type hypersensitivity is type 4 and is due to previously sensitized T lymphocytes, which release lymphokines upon reexposure to the antigen. This takes time—perhaps up to several days following exposure. The tuberculin reaction is the best known example of this. T cell–mediated cytotoxicity leads to lysis of cells by cytotoxic T cells in response to tumor cells, allogenic tissue, and virus-infected cells. These cells have CD8 antigens on their surfaces.

30. The answer is C. *(Anderson, ed 9. pp 209-213.)* Heavy metal poisoning may occur via the respiratory route owing to contaminated inhalant and vapors. Such poisoning is usually industrially related, as with mercury (calomel workers), arsenic (pesticides), and lead (batteries and paints). Cadmium has been implicated in producing not only an acute form of pneumonia, but, with chronic exposure to small concentrations of cadmium vapors, diffuse interstitial pulmonary fibrosis and an increased incidence of emphysema as well. The "honeycomb" radiologic pattern is indicative of an interstitial fibrotic process and may be the result of repeated pneumonitis and bronchitis. Cadmium can also be found in tobacco smoke. Cobalt poisoning leads to myocardiopathy, mercury poisoning leads to renal tubular damage, and lead poisoning leads to liver necrosis and cerebral edema. Arsenic poisoning, in addition to carrying an increased risk of lung and skin cancer, may produce death caused by inhibition of respiratory enzymes and cardiac subendocardial hemorrhages complicated by gastroenteritis with shock.

31. The answer is C. *(Anderson, ed 9. pp 531-532.)* An allograft is also called a homograft and refers to a graft between members of the same species. An autograft refers to a tissue graft taken from one site and placed in a different site in the same individual. Isografts are grafts between individuals from an inbred strain of animals. A graft between individuals of two different species is a xenograft or heterograft.

32. The answer is C. *(Robbins, ed 4. pp 207-209.)* Fifteen to twenty percent of cases of polymyositis are associated with underlying visceral malignancies of virtually any organ. Although the cause of this association remains unknown, it has been postulated that some cancers either produce products that are toxic to skeletal muscles or contain antigens that are cross-reactive with skeletal muscle.

33. The answer is D. *(Robbins, ed 4. pp 194-195, 205.)* Diagnostic specificity is defined as the probability of a negative diagnostic test result in the absence of the disease the test is designed to detect, or, simply, the ability of a screening test to correctly identify a person who is free of the specific disease. Two clinically useful tests specific for systemic lupus erythematosus (SLE) are the detection of antibodies to double-stranded DNA (anti-ds DNA) and to the nonhistone Smith (Sm) antigen, since these antibodies are rare in other autoimmune diseases. Positive testing for antinuclear antibody (ANA) occurs in virtually all patients with SLE (marked diagnostic sensitivity), but the test is *not specific* since positive results are frequent in other autoimmune diseases. In diffuse systemic sclerosis, positive antibodies to nucleolar RNA and Scl-70 antibody to nonhistone nuclear protein are specific. In the CREST syndrome of systemic sclerosis, an anticentromere antibody is specific. The best information from laboratory tests comes from their positive and negative predictive values (PVs) relating the results (+ or −) to prevalence of the disease in the population being studied.

34. The answer is B. *(Robbins, ed 4. pp 196-201.)* Renal failure is the most common cause of death in SLE. Most cases show some renal abnormality (mild or marked) by immunofluorescence and by light and electron microscopy. Diffuse proliferative glomerulonephritis (GN) occurs in about 50 percent of cases and is the most common and most serious renal lesion. Subendothelial location of immune complex deposits is particularly characteristic of SLE. Membranous GN occurs in only 10 percent of cases and has a better prognosis, but may progress. Polyclonal B-cell activation occurs with increased production of autoantibodies and hypergammaglobulinemia. This B-cell activation may follow genetic B-cell abnormalities or loss of T-suppressor cell influence. Most of the tissue lesions are mediated by the immune complex (type III hypersensitivity). Nonerosive arthritis occurs in about 90 percent of cases and often involves small peripheral joints. Lack of deformity and of synovial proliferation distinguish arthritis of SLE from rheumatoid arthritis.

35. The answer is C. *(Robbins, ed 4. pp 202-204.)* Sjögren's syndrome is characterized by dryness of the mouth (xerostomia) and eyes (keratoconjunctivitis sicca). Secondary Sjögren's syndrome is associated with rheumatoid arthritis (RA), or SLE, or systemic sclerosis. The primary form shows increased frequency of HLA-DR3, while association with RA shows a positive correlation with HLA-DR4. Anti-SSB antibodies are fairly specific, anti-SSA less so, and both may occur in SLE; rheumatoid factor is often present. Glomerular lesions are very rare but a mild tubulointerstitial nephritis is quite common and may result in renal tubular acidosis. In addition to the usual dense, lymphoplasmacytic infiltrate of salivary glands, the lymph nodes may show a "pseudolymphomatous" appearance. True B-cell lymphomas have developed with increased frequency in Sjögren's syndrome (relative risk of 44).

36. The answer is E. *(Robbins, ed 4. pp 183-188.)* Histocompatible antigens (HLA) are responsible for rejection of transplanted organs in humans. Organ rejection requires both humoral and cell-mediated immunologic reactions involving T cells both from the donated organ and the patient's own CD4 T helper cells and CD8 cytotoxic T cells. Hyperacute rejection occurs within minutes after transplantation and consists of neutrophils within the glomerulus and peritubular capillaries. Acute rejection occurs within days after transplantation and is marked by vasculitis and interstitial lymphocytic infiltration. Subacute rejection vasculitis occurs during the first few months after transplantation and is characterized by the proliferation of fibroblasts and macrophages in the tunica intima of arteries. In chronic rejection tubular atrophy, mononuclear interstitial infiltration, and vascular changes are encountered, with the vascular changes being characteristic and probably reflecting an end stage of arteritis. The vascular obliteration leads to interstitial fibrosis and tubular atrophy with loss of renal function. However, the histologic picture is complicated by secondary ischemic damage, and it may be difficult to discern inflammation, fibrosis, and vascular changes as cause or effect.

37. The answer is C. *(Robbins, ed 4. pp 366-367, 1355.)* A localized skin rash in the summertime followed within a period of weeks by arthritis, especially involving less than three joints, should arouse suspicion of Lyme disease. This disorder was first described in the mid 1970s in Connecticut when small clusters of cases of children suffering from an illness resembling juvenile rheumatoid arthritis were first noted. The disease has now been shown to be caused by a spirochete, *Borrelia burgdorferi*, through the bite of a tick belonging to the genus *Ixodes*. The spirochete-infested ticks reside in forested areas where there are deer and small rodents present. The deer act as a wintering-over reservoir for the ticks. In the spring the tick larval stage emerges and evolves into a nymph, which is infective for humans if they are bitten. Adult ticks are also capable of transmitting the spirochete as well during questing. The bite is followed by a rash called erythema chronicum migrans, which may resolve spontaneously. However, many patients have a transient phase of spirochetemia, which may allow the spread of the spirochete to the meninges, heart, and synovial tissue. Originally thought to be confined to New England, Lyme disease has now been shown to be present in Europe and in Australia as well. The spirochetes are sensitive to penicillin, erythromycin, and tetracycline. Reiter's disease does not present with a spreading rash, and a Baker's cyst produces swelling in the popliteal fossa behind the knee rather than joint effusions anteriorly.

38. The answer is C. *(Robbins, ed 4. p 1333.)* Hypertrophic osteoarthropathy is a syndrome consisting of periosteal new bone formation with, or without, digital clubbing and joint effusion. It is seen usually in an adult who complains of aching bone pain, especially in distal extremities. While it is most common in association with lung carcinoma (up to 10 percent of cases), it also occurs with pleural mesothelioma, chronic lung disease such as bronchiectasis or lung abscess, infective endocarditis, and, less commonly, with cirrhosis or inflammatory bowel disease (ulcerative colitis). It may occur with congenital heart, lung, or liver disease in children and in familial and idiopathic forms. Radiographs show periosteal thickening with new bone formation on diaphyseal ends of long bones. Treatment is that of the associated disorder, the arthropathy being reversible with surgical resection or medical correction of the underlying disease.

39. The answer is C. *(Anderson, ed 9. pp 1255-1256.)* Antibodies to mitochondria are not present in the serum of patients who have acute viral hepatitis when immunofluorescent techniques are used. Serum antibodies to mitochondria are present, however, in 87 percent of patients who have primary biliary cirrhosis, 69 percent of patients who have chlorpromazine-induced jaundice, 66 percent of patients who have chronic active hepatitis, and 18 percent of patients who have systemic lupus erythematosus. Immunofluorescent detection techniques for antibodies to mitochondria are not specific for one particular disease, but, when evaluated in conjunction with tests for antinuclear antibodies and antibodies to smooth muscle, they can be helpful in differential diagnosis.

40. The answer is D. *(Robbins, ed 4. pp 133-135.)* The Barr body represents a sex chromatin clump attached to the nuclear membrane that originates from an entire X chromosome and can easily be seen by using light microscopy to examine scrapings of the epithelium of the inside buccal mucosa. According to the formula M = $n - 1$, the total number of X chromatin masses equals the number of cellular X chromatin masses seen in the nucleus minus 1. Hence, normal males are $0 = 1 - 1$ (no Barr body), and normal females are $1 = 2 - 1$ (one Barr body). In classic Turner's syndrome (XO), the expected buccal smear would be $0 = 1 - 1$ (no Barr bodies seen), as in a normal male. Karyotyping is necessary when the Barr body screening test is ambiguous or inconclusive. In a young woman of short stature and average intelligence who has never menstruated, there is a strong indication that one of the forms of Turner's syndrome exists, and the presence of one Barr body indicates that the patient has XX in some percentage of cells. About 10 percent of all Turner's syndrome patients show a mosaic pattern, with some cells having XO/XX or XO/XXX patterns. In this example, the patient is likely to be XO/XX by the formula $1 = 2 - 1$. In Turner's mosaics, the likelihood of developing a seminoma or gonadoblastoma is higher than expected, and gonadectomy may be indicated.

41. The answer is A. *(Henry, ed 17. pp 212-213.)* C-reactive protein (CRP) elevations, as well as elevations in the erythrocyte sedimentation rate, are nonspecific markers of inflammatory conditions. The CRP rises faster and returns to normal earlier than the erythrocyte sedimentation rate in most inflammatory diseases. Most bacterial infections, rheumatoid arthritis, rheumatic fever, and diseases leading to necrosis and tissue damage will elevate the CRP. CRP elevations do not occur in most viral illnesses.

42. The answer is C. *(Robbins, ed 4. p 369.)* Although the rapid plasma reagin (RPR) test, Kolmer test, and Veneral Disease Research Laboratory (VDRL) test are rapid and easily performed tests that can help confirm a diagnosis of active syphilis, these tests, because of their low specificity for antibodies against treponemal or cardiolipin antigens, are associated with false-positive reactions. Therefore, RPR tests, Kolmer tests, and VDRL tests usually are used for screening programs. The *Treponema pallidum* immobilization (TPI) test and the fluorescent treponemal antibody-absorption (FTA-ABS) test have greater specificity for treponemal antigen but are technically more difficult to perform. The FTA-ABS test is generally the most sensitive and most specific of the syphilis testing procedures.

43. The answer is E. *(Robbins, ed 4. pp 380-382.)* Lepromatous and tuberculoid leprosy, the major forms, are caused by *Mycobacterium leprae* and nerve involvement is most typical of the lepromatous form. Numerous bacilli in packets occupy histiocytes or lepra cells in the lesions of lepromatous leprosy. Polyclonal hypergammaglobulinemia often occurs in lepromatous leprosy, in which patients do not have the adequate cellular immune response of the tuberculoid form. Large amounts of anti-lepra antibody occur in the lepromatous form with frequent formation of antigen-antibody complexes and resultant disorders such as erythema nodosum. A "clear" zone between infiltrate and overlying epidermis is characteristic of lepromatous leprosy, unlike the encroachment on basal epidermis of the tuberculoid infiltrate.

44. The answer is D. *(Anderson, ed 9. pp 2-3.)* The cytoplasmic matrix contains numerous organelles with highly specialized functions. Whereas mitochondria are the "power" units of the cell involved with the Krebs cycle and anaerobic metabolism, the endoplasmic reticulum is a complex network of rodlike tubules containing ribosomes and is involved in protein synthesis (rough endoplasmic reticulum). Lysosomes are round bodies containing enzymes involved in inflammation. These include the sulfatases, desoxyribonucleases, hydrolases, and acid phosphatates. The Golgi apparatus (complex) is made up of tiny vesicles, membranes, and vacuoles and is also involved in protein synthesis, as it receives the synthesized proteins from the endoplasmic reticulum. The Golgi complex appears to collect, segregate, and export protein. Microbodies are membrane-bound spheres that contain catalase, oxidases, and uric acid oxidase. Epithelial cells, especially surface-lining cells, are held together by connections referred to as intercellular junctions. Desmosomes (squamous cells), tight junctions (zonula occludens), and gap junctions (nexuses) are examples of such membrane connectors.

45. The answer is E. *(Robbins, ed 4. pp 365-366, 372.)* Lymphogranuloma venereum, usually transmitted by sexual contact, is caused by obligate intracellular parasites that contain both RNA and DNA and belong to the genus *Chlamydia (C. trachomatis).* Chlamydial agents, originally thought to be viruses because they form inclusion bodies in infected cells, also cause trachoma, inclusion conjunctivitis, and psittacosis-ornithosis. The other infections listed are caused by spirochetes and are nonvenereal.

46. The answer is E. *(Henry, ed 17. p 947.)* Elevations in cerebrospinal fluid globulins often occur in multiple sclerosis and other demyelinating diseases. An abnormal band on electrophoresis may occur even in the absence of elevated globulins. Late tertiary syphilis may cause these findings, but they would not occur in the secondary stage. Tumor or meningeal leukemia can also produce elevated levels of globulin in cerebrospinal fluid, but the presence of tumor cells and absence of an electrophoretic band would lead to the proper diagnosis.

47. The answer is A. *(Henry, ed 17. p 497.)* Although human chorionic gonadotropin (HCG) levels characteristically are elevated in all the conditions listed, up to 50 percent of patients with an ectopic pregnancy may have urine levels of HCG less than 1.0 IU/ml. Since many of the pregnancy tests used do not detect levels in this range, a negative test for urinary HCG does not rule out an ectopic pregnancy.

48. The answer is A. *(Robbins, ed 4. p 240.)* All tumors whether benign or malignant have a supporting stroma composed of varying amounts of connective tissue and blood supply. The cellularity can range from that of a highly cellular lesion, such as oat cell carcinoma of the lung or Burkitt's lymphoma, to that of a relatively hypocellular lesion, such as a hyalinized neurilemmoma, but the cellularity of the tumor per se does not usually influence the texture. Firmness and even hardness of tumors are a function of the amount of collagenous stroma present. The term *desmoplasia* refers to a collagenized and fibroblastic stroma; an example is carcinoma of the breast, which has the texture of a water chestnut because of the concurrent proliferation of the fibrous stroma with the carcinoma. Tumors that lack a collagenized fibrous stroma tend to be softer regardless of the tumor cellularity per se. Malignant tumors of mesenchyme have a fleshy character because of very little connective tissue stroma; examples include fibrosarcoma, liposarcoma, and leiomyosarcoma. There are a few exceptions to the desmoplastic rule, and an obvious example is a tumor of cartilage in which the hyaline cartilage matrix accounts for the firmness; some chondrosarcomas, however, may be soft and friable.

49. The answer is B. *(Robbins, ed 4. pp 695, 1070.)* A fulminating septic state should always be considered and excluded whenever the constellation of fever, deteriorating mental status, skin hemorrhages, and shock develops. Such conditions can be seen in gram-negative rod septicemia caused by any of the coliforms (gram-negative endotoxic shock) or fulminant meningococcemia (Waterhouse-Friderichsen syndrome). However, a form of nonbacterial vasculitis termed thrombotic thrombocytopenic purpura (TTP) is notorious for producing a clinical syndrome very similar to fulminating infective states. It is characterized by arteriole and capillary occlusions by fibrin and platelet microthrombi and is usually unassociated with any of the predisposing states seen in disseminated intravascular coagulopathy (DIC), such as malignancy, infection, retained fetus, and amniotic fluid embolism. Macrocytic hemolytic anemia, variable jaundice, renal failure, skin hemorrhages, and central nervous system dysfunction are all seen in TTP and are related to the fibrin thrombi, which can be demonstrated with skin, bone marrow, and lymph node biopsies. The vasculitis usually shows no inflammatory cells, which distinguishes TTP from other forms of vasculitis. There is less coagulopathy in TTP than is found in DIC, and hemolytic anemia is generally not found in idiopathic or autoimmune thrombocytopenic purpura. The condition of patients with TTP may be temporarily improved by plasmapheresis, but the outcome is usually grim.

50. The answer is C. *(Henry, ed 17. p 126.)* The type of blood sample sent to the laboratory, the type of container used to collect blood, the manner in which the blood specimen was collected, and the preparation of the patient (appropriate fasting, drug history, exercise) prior to venipuncture are just as important to the final laboratory result as the analytic method used by the laboratory to arrive at the result. All these factors can cause deviations in laboratory results, and they should be considered before accepting abnormal laboratory results. Red blood cells can readily lyse because of alcohol left on the arm while swabbing the skin, use of unclean or poorly dried syringes or too large a needle bore (17 gauge, for example), or a traumatic venipuncture. Since red blood cells contain a higher concentration of K^+ than does serum or plasma, even moderate hemolysis of red cells can cause spurious elevation of serum K^+. If the serum clot tube is seen to be slightly pink, most laboratories will notify the ward that an improper sample has been obtained. Once the laboratory result is confirmed as being valid, the next step is to exclude intravascular hemolysis within the patient before making a diagnosis of hyperkalemia.

51. The answer is C. *(Henry, ed 17. p 147. Robbins, ed 4. pp 1242–1243.)* Parathyroid hormone (PTH), by affecting the kidneys, bones, and intestinal mucosa, is the principal regulator of plasma levels of phosphate and calcium. PTH, by its action on renal tubular cells, not only causes decreased phosphate reabsorption, it causes increased calcium reabsorption; these reciprocal processes result in a decrease in serum phosphate and a corresponding increase in extracellular calcium levels. Extracellular levels of calcium are also maintained by the release of calcium during PTH-induced osteocytic and osteoclastic osteolysis, a process that is regarded as the mobilization of calcium from bone. PTH also may induce the intestinal mucosa to absorb calcium derived from dietary sources.

52. The answer is A. *(Henry, ed 17. pp 263-264, 275-277.)* Serum glutamic-oxaloacetic transaminase (SGOT) levels (curve II) become elevated within 12 hours after nearly all acute myocardial infarctions; they generally reach a peak level within 48 hours and return to normal within 4 to 5 days. After myocardial infarctions, creatine phosphokinase levels (curve I) rise and fall more rapidly than do SGOT levels. Lactic dehydrogenase levels (curve III) also become elevated within 1 day after infarctions, but they remain elevated for about 10 days. Alkaline phosphatase and 5'-nucleotidase levels, normal during infarctions, usually show marked increases in patients who have obstructive jaundice.

53. The answer is D. *(Henry, ed 17. pp 37-38, 394.)* Although most laboratories are capable of directly measuring the serum or urine osmolality with accurate osmometers, it is useful to remember the following formula:

$$\text{Osmolality (mOsm/kg) } H_2O = 2 \times [Na^+] + \frac{[\text{glucose}]}{20} + \frac{[\text{BUN}]}{3}$$

This formula gives an approximation of the serum osmolality in a given patient, since Na^+, glucose, and blood urea nitrogen account for at least 95 percent of the dissolved solutes composing the osmolality. The normal serum osmolality falls within the range of 285 to 310 mOsm/kg H_2O. An often overlooked cause of profound water loss with dehydration (in osmotic diseases) in elderly diabetic patients is nonketotic, hyperosmolar coma. These patients enter a phase of coma and dehydration with vascular collapse owing to hypovolemia caused by profound osmotic diuresis that is in turn due to the striking hyperglycemia. The serum acetoacetic acid and ketone levels may be normal or mildly elevated in contrast to the ketoacidosis of diabetic coma in younger patients.

54. The answer is E. *(Robbins, ed 4. pp 450-452.)* Thiamine (vitamin B_1) deficiency causes beriberi and occurs in populations with diets of polished rice or milled grains because of the loss of the high thiamine content of discarded husks. Enzymatic degradation of thiamine by thiaminases in raw fish, shellfish, or meat occurs, so that a diet of mainly raw food may cause beriberi. Alcoholism is a major cause, owing to decreased thiamine intake with poor general nutrition and further loss from vomiting and ethanol-induced diuresis. Deficiencies may also result with diuretic therapy because of increased loss of the water-soluble vitamin. Scurvy (deficiency of vitamin C) is closely associated with a diet low in fruits and vegetables.

55. The answer is D. *(Grizzle, Arch Pathol Lab Med 113:727-728, 1989.)* In Cushing's syndrome diagnostic laboratory tests have improved from relatively nonspecific urinary assays of 17-ketogenic steroids and 17-hydroxycorticosteroids to more specific radioimmunoassays measuring ACTH, corticotropin releasing factor (CRF), cortisol, and other plasma steroids as well as urinary free cortisol—a reliable, cost-effective screening method. After diagnosis of Cushing's syndrome, its cause must be identified by the dexamethasone (synthetic analogue of cortisol) high-dose suppression test, reliable ACTH radioimmunoassays, and imaging techniques of computed tomography (sella turcica) and nuclear magnetic resonance. Small pituitary microadenomas may be identified now by selective venous sampling for ACTH and other peptides from the inferior petrosal sinuses draining the pituitary. Plasma cortisol levels fluctuate rather widely and the urinary 17-ketosteroids give information about androgen metabolites, not about glucocorticoid activity.

56. The answer is A. *(Henry, ed 17. pp 538-539.)* Low levels of serum amylase usually are found in patients who have diabetes mellitus, congestive heart failure, gastrointestinal cancer or obstruction, fractures, or pleurisy. High levels of serum amylase usually are found in patients who have mumps, renal insufficiency, or ruptured ectopic pregnancy; who have received morphine; or who develop obstruction, strangulation, or perforation complications after abdominal surgery.

57. The answer is A. *(Henry, ed 17. pp 135-136.)* The renal plasma clearance of any substance (X) is expressed as the volume of plasma from which X is removed by renal activity per unit of time, usually 1 minute. In the clearance formula shown below, U_x represents the concentration of X in milligrams per milliliter of urine; V represents urine volume per minute and usually is derived from a 24-hour urine volume; P_x represents the plasma concentration of X in milligrams per milliliter; and C_x represents the volume of plasma cleared of substance X per minute.

$$C_x = \frac{(U_x)(V)}{P_x}$$

By interpolation of the given data into appropriate units and by substitution, the equation becomes

$$C_x = \frac{(0.469 \text{ mg/ml})(0.535 \text{ ml/min})}{0.02 \text{ mg/ml}}$$

The answer is 12.5 ml/min. For males, normal creatinine clearance values range from 107 to 139 ml/min; for females, the range is 87 to 107 ml/min.

58. The answer is C. *(Bullough, pp 5.4-5.8.)* Hyperuricemia, prominent in gout, occurs most often secondary to disorders that increase production or reduce excretion of uric acid. These include myeloproliferative disorders and some cancers in which there is increased turnover of nucleic acid, with resultant hyperuricemia. Reduced excretion of uric acid may arise from renal causes, or from competition by certain organic acids, as in starvation ketosis. Chondrocalcinosis, or calcium pyrophosphate dihydrate (CPPD) deposition disease, is not associated with hyperuricemia.

59. The answer is A. *(Robbins, ed 4. pp 323-325.)* If bilirubinuria and pyridium therapy are excluded, the presence of pink-orange-brown casts with contained granular debris or intact red cells within the casts always implies the presence of significant glomerular damage, usually in the form of immune complex glomerulonephritis (poststreptococcal, lupus, Goodpasture's) or owing to renal infarction. Damage to the glomerular capillary loops or the basement membrane allows the leakage of red cells and protein, which condense into casts in the distal tubules, are subsequently passed into the urine, and become directly visible under the microscope in urinalysis. Whereas renal biopsies are usually necessary to categorize the nature of the glomerulonephritis completely, poststreptococcal glomerulonephritis may be implicated if the antistreptolysin titer (ASO titer) or anti-DNase-B titers are elevated.

60. The answer is B. *(Robbins, ed 4. pp 243-250.)* As all medical oncologists and students of oncology are painfully aware, tumors do not read textbooks and cannot be expected to follow predicted courses in every clinical circumstance. Thus, many exceptions and deviations from the expected occur. An important predictor of a given tumor's behavior, however, is the differentiation, which is a histologic parameter that gives some index as to the degree of resemblance of the tumor to the cell of origin; that is, differentiation states to what degree the tumor resembles its parent cell or tissues. Well-differentiated tumors resemble their cells of origin to a great extent, while poorly differentiated tumors do not resemble their origins to an appreciable extent. With some exceptions tumors may be expected to behave according to their differentiation. Furthermore, the growth rate of tumors appears to correlate with their level of differentiation, with the less-differentiated tumors growing faster than well-differentiated ones. The term *grade* implies differentiation and in some cases may be synonymous; for example, grade I tumors are well differentiated, while grade III tumors are poorly differentiated. Higher grade tumors tend to have more mitoses, which generally correlate with aggressiveness and final outcome.

61. The answer is E. *(Henry, ed 17. pp 260–262.)* Normal alkaline phosphatase levels are common in patients who have myocardial infarctions. Elevated levels of this nonlipid esterase are usually demonstrable in patients who have hepatitis, infectious mononucleosis, cirrhosis, or obstructive jaundice. In polycythemia vera, marked elevation of alkaline phosphatase is considered a classic sign and has been demonstrated in 80 percent of cases of this myeloproliferative syndrome.

62. The answer is C. *(Henry, ed 17. pp 775-777.)* Von Willebrand's disease is not as rare as once thought, and numerous subtypes, which are delineated by two-dimensional electrophoresis, have been described. The disease is characterized clinically by mucocutaneous bleeding, menorrhagia, and epistaxis. Milder forms of the disease may not be diagnosed until the patient is older. Factor VIII is a complex of several components that can be discerned electrophoretically. Of all the factor VIII components, factor VIII:R, or ristocetin cofactor, is most apt to be abnormal in von Willebrand's disease. The coagulant (C) and the related antigen (Ag) forms of factor VIII may sometimes be normal in various autosomal dominant types. Most patients even with the milder forms will have decreased factor VIII:R. Prothrombin time and fibrinogen levels are not affected in this disorder.

63. The answer is A. *(Henry, ed 17. pp 236-237.)* The patient described probably has hepatitis, according to the values given for the five isoenzymes of lactic dehydrogenase (LDH). Liver cells contain higher proportions of LDH_4 and LDH_5 than do myocardium or red blood cells, both of which contain greater relative amounts of LDH_1 and LDH_2. Lung tissue is high in LDH_3, and brain tissue contains only small amounts of LDH_5.

64. The answer is B. *(Robbins, ed 4. pp 253, 261, 288, 715-716, 718.)* Burkitt's lymphoma is one of the most rapidly growing tumors known to oncologists. Most tumors grow without inhibition by means of a decrease in the time spent within the cell growth cycle itself, a reduction in the total numbers of cells dying, or many more stable cells leaving G_0 to enter the cycle at G_1. One or all of these mechanisms may be in effect, along with a lack of inhibition of cell growth. Such inhibition is not completely understood, but cells are known to be delayed in progressing to mitosis from G_2. Permanent cells are essentially nondividing and usually die. In African Burkitt's lymphoma, but not necessarily in American Burkitt's lymphoma, high titers of serum antibody to Epstein-Barr viral capsid antigen have been described, along with incorporation of the viral genome. A translocation occurs between chromosome 8 (site of proto-oncogene c-myc) and chromosome 14, which carries the heavy-chain Ig gene, t (8; 14).

65. The answer is D. *(Robbins, ed 4. pp 269, 272.)* The association of the chemical and physical environment (with its implied hazards of toxic wastes, mainly from industrial pollution) with the development of tumors in humans is becoming a specialized field in itself. Major legislation and public health efforts are just beginning to place emphasis on these hazards. A major clue to the implication of environmental factors lies in the clustering of rare tumor types in populations in which such an incidence is unexpected. For example, cases of angiosarcoma of the liver (a relatively rare tumor) were identified in employees of a rubber company and in a few residents living near the plant where the monomer vinyl chloride was present in the atmosphere. Exposure to asbestos in shipyard, roofing, and insulation workers has led to the development of not only pleural and peritoneal malignant mesotheliomas, but solid malignant tumors of the lung and viscera as well. Although it increases the risk of tuberculosis, silicosis has not, by itself, increased the risk of developing cancer. Similarly, beryllium vapor (from the manufacture of alloys, ceramics, high-technology electronics, and fluorescent light bulbs) causes marked granulomatous disease but has not been identified as a carcinogen. Cyanide is lethal if ingested. Carbon tetrachloride and chloroform may cause hepatic necrosis and are potentially lethal, but neither is implicated in tumorigenesis. Foundry workers are at risk of developing pulmonary and nasal sinus cancers when they are regularly exposed to nickel or chromium compounds.

66. The answer is D. *(Henry, ed 17. pp 305-307.)* Triiodothyronine (T_3) is the thyroid hormone with the greatest physiologic activity, although thyroxine (T_4) is present in greater quantities and thus is usually the best measure of thyroid activity. Monoiodotyrosine (MIT) and diiodotyrosine (DIT) are not released from the gland and have little activity. Thyroglobulin is the carrier protein for binding stored thyroid hormones.

67. The answer is C. *(Robbins, ed 4. pp 1260-1261.)* A tendency to lose salt and water often appears in adrenogenital syndrome with adrenocortical hyperplasia. There is general agreement that in the salt-losing form of this syndrome aldosterol and cortisol production is deficient, a consequence of genetically impaired biosynthesis of adrenal corticoids. Adrenogenital syndrome also may be known as "congenital virilizing adrenocortical hyperplasia," a generic term that probably should be discarded because it paradoxically includes forms not associated with virilization.

68. The answer is B. *(Anderson, ed 9. pp 52-53.)* Tay-Sachs disease (G_{M2} gangliosidosis type 1), first recognized in 1881 by Warren Tay, is a storage disease in which the G_{M2} ganglioside accumulates in neurons because of a deficiency in β-N-acetylhexosaminidase. The G_{M2} ganglioside structurally lacks a terminal galactose unit. Tay-Sachs disease, the major form of gangliosidosis, afflicts thousands of patients. Major clinical features of Tay-Sachs disease include macrocephaly caused by cerebral gliosis, mental-motor deterioration, and lipidosis of cortical, autonomic, and rectal mucosal neurons.

69. The answer is A. *(Robbins, ed 4. pp 146, 154.)* Fabry's disease, first described by Anderson and Fabry independently, may be hemizygous or heterozygous and is caused by a deficiency in α-galactosidase A, which leads to abnormal accumulations of glycosphingolipid (trihexosylceramide) within the lysosomes of vascular-endothelial and smooth muscle cells of the heart and kidney, ganglion cells, and epithelial cells of the cornea. Multiple angiokeratomata of the skin in a patient with tortuous conjunctival vessels and corneal opacity are highly suggestive of the disease. Death usually ensues from progressive renal failure and uremia. Birefringent lipid bodies (Maltese crosses) may be seen in the urine sediment with polarized light.

70. The answer is C. *(Robbins, ed 4. p 127.)* Any deviation from the normal number of chromosomes, from their normal structure, or any combination of the two is an aberration that, if unbalanced, is termed *aneuploidy*. If the alterations remain balanced (balanced translocations), the condition is termed *euploidy*. Aneuploidy can result from the addition of a single chromosome to a pair (trisomy) from translocations, inversions, duplications, and deletions.

71. The answer is A. *(Braunwald, ed 11. pp 1208-1209.)* Renal tubular acidosis (RTA) can be either due to a gradient defect (the classic form) or due to bicarbonate wastage. In the classic form of this syndrome, too many hydrogen ions diffuse back from tubular urine to blood. This "back-diffusion" occurs in the distal tubules and prevents the formation of a steep pH gradient between blood and tubular urine.

Ammonia excretion is normal in both forms of RTA. In RTA caused by bicarbonate wastage, the depressed reabsorption of bicarbonate ions in the proximal tubules leads to the spillage of these ions into urine.

72. The answer is D. *(Robbins, ed 4. pp 342, 782.)* Most cases of lobar pneumonia are caused by *Streptococcus pneumoniae* (reclassification of the pneumococcus). Streptococcal or pneumococcal pneumonia involves one or more lobes and is often seen in alcoholics or debilitated persons. Type 3 pneumococcus (*S. pneumoniae*) causes a virulent lobar pneumonia characterized by mucoid sputum, which is also seen in *Klebsiella* pneumonia. *K. pneumoniae* (Friedländer's bacillus) usually produces a bronchopneumonia, rather than lobar pneumonia, but is clinically indistinguishable from pneumococcal lobar pneumonia. *Legionella* species cause a fibrinopurulent lobular pneumonia that tends to be confluent, almost appearing lobar.

73. The answer is A. *(Robbins, ed 4. pp 334, 342.)* The rough or unencapsulated strains of *Streptococcus (Diplococcus) pneumoniae* are not thought to be pathogenic for humans. A capsule protects the bacteria and confers pathogenicity; the degree of virulence varies among antigenic types. Testing encapsulated species (e.g., type 3) with the appropriate antiserum leads to a positive quellung test (capsular swelling or refractivity).

74. The answer is D. *(Robbins, ed 4. pp 165-167.)* B cells possess surface membrane IgM and IgD, with monomeric IgM the antigen receptor of all B cells. B cells also express the pan–B-cell antigens CD19 and CD20, which is obviously of practical value in differentiating a chronic leukemia such as chronic lymphocytic leukemia (CLL) in which transformed B cells possess surface IgM and IgD and express CD19 and CD20 antigens, but not the early B cell antigen CD10. In contrast, CD8 and CD4 are on 30 percent and 60 percent of peripheral T cells, respectively. CD4 is a marker for T helper cells, and CD8 a marker for cytotoxic/suppressor T cells. B lymphocytes have receptors for fixed complement components C3b and C3d and for the Fc portion of IgG. Immunologic diagnosis of B-cell lymphoid tumors by immunofluorescence or flow cytometry shows the cell surface immunoglobulins and cluster differentiation antigens through detection by monoclonal antibodies; molecular biology techniques reveal Ig gene rearrangements on the altered B cells.

75. The answer is D. *(Robbins, ed 4. pp 357-358.)* *Yersinia* (formerly called *Pasteurella*) is an important genus of gram-negative bacilli that cause a wide variety of human and animal disease, ranging from plague (*Y. pestis*) to acute mesenteric lymphadenitis (*Y. enterocolitica*) in older children and young adults. *Y. enterocolitica* infections also occur in the terminal ileum in young adults, causing an ileitis that produces inflammation not unlike that seen in some stages of Crohn's disease (regional enteritis). Since the organisms grow slowly on enrichment media, they may be overgrown by other coliforms at 37°C. The organisms may be isolated by means of cold enhancement at 4°C.

76. The answer is C. *(Robbins, ed 4. pp 386-387, 393-394.)* In the approximate center of the photomicrograph is the classic, refractile, double-walled spherule of the deep fungus *Coccidioides immitis,* which is several times the diameter of the largest inflammatory cell nearby. Coccidioidomycosis is endemic in California, Arizona, New Mexico, and parts of Nevada, Utah, and Texas, where it resides in the arid soils and is contracted by direct inhalation of airborne dust. If inhaled, it produces a primary pulmonary infection that is usually benign and self-limiting in immunologically competent persons, often with several days of fever and upper respiratory flulike symptoms. However, certain ethnic groups, such as some blacks, Asians, and Filipinos, are at risk of developing a potentially lethal disseminated form of the disease that can involve the central nervous system. If the large, double-walled spherule containing numerous endospores can be demonstrated outside the lungs (e.g., in a skin biopsy), this is evidence of dissemination. Antibodies of high titers are detectable by means of complement fixation studies in patients undergoing spontaneous recovery. Amphotericin B is usually reserved for treating high-risk and disseminated infection. The cultured mycelia of the organism on Sabouraud's agar present a hazard for laboratory workers.

77. The answer is B. *(Robbins, ed 4. pp 182-183.)* Delayed-hypersensitivity reactions are mediated by T lymphocytes and other mononuclear cells. The reaction requires previous exposure to antigen, frequently a large protein, and takes from 1 to 3 days to develop fully. Only true palpable induration is considered a positive reaction.

78. The answer is A. *(Robbins, ed 4. pp 178-180.)* Serum sickness is associated with antigen-antibody complexes produced and cleared in an environment of antigen excess. The complexes induce focal vascular lesions in many arterial and capillary beds. The other "allergic" responses listed in the question are associated with much smaller amounts of antigen.

79. The answer is C. *(Robbins, ed 4. pp 373-375.)* Pathogenic mycobacteria, including *M. tuberculosis,* have a known propensity for resistance to drying in the environment, survival for extended periods of time on inanimate surfaces, resistance to alkali and acids, and impermeability to routine tissue and Gram stains. Many of these features are thought to be related to the very high lipid and wax content of the bacilli, which makes up some 60 percent of the total dry weight. Mycolic acid is only one of many fatty acids present. Virulence is thought to be related to the presence of the mycoside trehalose 6-6 dimycolate (cord factor).

80. The answer is A. *(Robbins, ed 4. pp 312-315, 320, 325.)* Togaviruses, a family of helical, predominantly single-stranded RNA viruses, include dengue and yellow fever viruses (both associated with hemorrhagic fever) and eastern, western, and St. Louis encephalitis viruses. These are all arthropod-borne. The causative agent of epidemic hemorrhagic keratoconjunctivitis is usually the type B adenovirus, an icosahedral double-stranded DNA virus. Herpes simplex keratoconjunctivitis, although frequently recurrent, is not epidemic.

81. The answer is E. *(Robbins, ed 4. pp 374-375.) Mycobacterium tuberculosis* is an obligate aerobe—thus its predilection for pulmonary infection. The high content of lipids in its cell wall is in part responsible for its acid-fast response to Ziehl-Neelsen staining. The frequency of occurrence of drug-resistant mutants in this organism has necessitated simultaneous use of multiple chemotherapeutic agents against it. Persons with silicosis have a high incidence of infection with *M. tuberculosis*, which on culture requires several weeks to grow.

82. The answer is D. *(Robbins, ed 4. pp 386-387, 390-391.) Cryptococcus neoformans* is a true pathogen. It is not dimorphic, as are *Coccidioides immitis*, *Histoplasma capsulatum*, and *Blastomyces dermatitidis*. *Aspergillus fumigatus* is also not dimorphic but grows as a mycelium and not as an encapsulated yeast. All the organisms listed in the question can cause systemic disease, but except for *C. neoformans*, respiratory involvement is the major clinical problem they cause. Although *C. neoformans* usually enters via the lung, pulmonary involvement is often minimal, and the meningeal involvement is the most serious common aspect of infection.

83. The answer is E. *(Robbins, ed 4. pp 333-334, 784-785.) Mycoplasma pneumoniae*, the causative agent of primary atypical interstitial pneumonia, belongs to the mycoplasma group of tiny pleuropneumonia-like organisms (PPLOs, or Eaton agents), which lack cell walls and are beyond the resolution of light microscopy. *M. pneumoniae* can cause up to 50 percent of pneumonias in college students and mainly affects adolescents and young adults. The interstitial pneumonia with mononuclear response is similar to viral pneumonia; pharyngitis and tracheobronchitis with persistent cough are common. Serum immunoglobulins that agglutinate human type O red cells at 4°C (cold agglutinins) are often present; this test is nonspecific, but suggestive of *M. pneumoniae*.

84. The answer is C. *(Robbins, ed 4. pp 318-324.)* Influenza is caused by small RNA viruses, classified as myxoviruses. All the other viral illnesses listed in the question are caused by herpesviruses, which are relatively large, double-stranded DNA viruses. Shingles and chickenpox are caused by herpes zoster, which is identical to varicella. Cytomegalovirus causes cytomegalic inclusion disease, and Epstein-Barr (EB) virus causes mononucleosis.

85. The answer is C. *(Robbins, ed 4. pp 488-489.)* Despite current controversy, most researchers agree that women taking oral contraceptives are at risk, however small, of developing myocardial infarction, especially if the woman is a cigarette smoker, and vascular thrombi that may lead to strokes and pulmonary embolism and infarction. Also very minimal in terms of numbers of cases are hepatic adenomas, which have been recorded in patients taking oral estrogens over a protracted period of time. Conflicting evidence is found concerning the risk of developing endometrial carcinoma. Some researchers have shown a definite risk of developing uterine cancer, but not all series have demonstrated a positive correlation. The same problem exists in estimation of the risk of developing breast cancer. Vaginal adenosis develops not in the women taking estrogens themselves, but rather in the female offspring of mothers who received diethylstilbestrol (DES) while pregnant. Some of these daughters have also developed clear cell carcinoma of the cervix, an adenocarcinoma that carries a rather poor prognosis. DES binds to cell nuclear DNA and hence may act as a cocarcinogen rather than as a mere promoter.

86. The answer is D. *(Robbins, ed 4. pp 490-492.)* The seemingly innumerable deleterious effects of alcohol abuse are recognized as constituting a major public health problem even in non-Western locations, such as Africa and Asia. The effects may be socioeconomic (divorce, absenteeism, and high insurance rates due to automobile accidents), political, moral, or organic. Indeed, it is difficult to think of an organ or organ system that does not develop a physical dysfunction, either reversible or irreversible, in response to excessive intake of ethanol. Subdural hematomas are commonly seen in alcoholics. Portal vein thrombosis is rarely seen in the absence of nutritional or Laennec's cirrhosis. Levels of the muscle and cardiac enzyme creatine phosphokinase may be elevated in states of alcoholic myocardiosis, cardiomyopathy, alcoholic rhabdomyolysis, or trauma to skeletal muscles while the patient is in an alcoholic toxic state. Primary biliary cirrhosis occurs predominantly in middle-aged women and its etiology is unknown, although marked immunologic factors have been described, as well as marked copper deposition in the liver, with normal serum ceruloplasmin.

87. The answer is C. *(Robbins, ed 4. p 362.)* Listeriosis is a food-borne illness (e.g., via milk products, coleslaw) usually occurring in the immunocompromised, in pregnant women and their fetuses, and in the debilitated elderly. *Listeria monocytogenes* is a gram-positive motile bacillus, often found within circulating lymphocytes (similar to *Legionella*). Maternal infection is mild; fetal infection is severe. Meningitis is predominant in neonatal infections and in opportunistic adult disease, and *Listeria monocytogenes* is responsible for about 2 percent of bacterial meningitis cases in this country. True epithelioid granulomas are rare, although macrophages may appear late, following neutrophil infiltration or abscesses in organs or lymph nodes.

88. The answer is D. *(Braunwald, ed 11. pp 1392-1396.)* AIDS is caused by infection with the retrovirus human immunodeficiency virus (HIV) (formerly called HTLV III/LAV). The virus infects T helper cells, preventing function, destroying cells, and increasing susceptibility to and incidence of infection. Cytotoxic/suppressor T cells may be normal, slightly increased, or decreased in number, although they show a proportional increase in comparison to helper T cells, which are markedly decreased. In AIDS, the ratio of helper to suppressor cells is inverted, being approximately 1:2, instead of the normal 2:1. Wide defects of immune function in AIDS include defects in natural killer cells, in monocytes, and in virus-specific cytotoxic T cells and B cells. B cells are polyclonally activated, resulting in hypergammaglobulinemia. Histologic diagnosis of chronic lymphoid interstitial pneumonitis in a child under 13 years of age is indicative of AIDS unless tests for HIV are negative.

89. The answer is A (1, 2, 3). *(Robbins, ed 4. pp 798-801, 874.)* Small-cell (oat cell) carcinoma of the lung occurs in 80 to 85 percent of cases of lung carcinoma in cigarette smokers and is populated by a cell that is characterized by endocrine-like features. Ultrastructurally, the cytoplasm contains neurosecretory granules similar to other cells of the APUD system—e.g., carcinoid and Kultschitzky cells, which are associated with the elaboration of hormones and enzymes such as ACTH, calcitonin, histaminase, serotonin, ADH, and L dopa decarboxylase. Owing to the release of substances into the circulation, endocrine-like syndromes are manifested symptomatically. For example, if the tumor secretes ACTH, the patient becomes frankly cushingoid. Other tumors produce ADH, which causes hyponatremia owing to vascular volume expansion (syndrome of inappropriate ADH). Elaboration of parathormone or parathormone-like hormones in lung carcinoma, with consequent hypercalcemia, is usually associated with squamous carcinoma of the lung rather than oat cell carcinoma. The carcinoid syndrome, complete with episodic facial flushing, vasomotor responses, and bronchoconstriction, has been identified in oat cell carcinoma and is due to the release of biogenic amines, such as serotonin.

90. The answer is A (1, 2, 3). *(Robbins, ed 4. pp 441-447.)* Vitamin D is essential for maintenance of normal bone remodeling in the adult; therefore, a significant deficiency in adults leads to poorly mineralized bone, or osteomalacia. Deficiency also results in decreased intestinal absorption of calcium, inadequate serum calcium and phosphorus, and, therefore, impaired mineralization of osteoid. Defective mineralization of osteoid causes formation of soft, easily deformed bones. Since there is no decreased production of osteoid matrix, a relative excess of woven bone or osteoid with wide osteoid seams results.

91. The answer is A (1, 2, 3). *(Robbins, ed 4. pp 65-68.)* Granulomatous inflammation is characterized by the presence of granulomas, consisting of 1- to 2-mm foci of modified macrophages (epithelioid cells) surrounded by mononuclear cells, mainly lymphocytes. It is a chronic inflammation initiated by a variety of infectious and noninfectious agents. Indigestible organisms or particles, or T-cell–mediated immunity to the inciting agent, or both, appear essential for formation of granulomas.

Although tuberculosis is the classic infectious granulomatous disease, several other infectious disorders are characterized by formation of granulomas, including deep fungal infections (coccidioidomycosis and histoplasmosis), schistosomiasis, syphilis, brucellosis, lymphogranuloma venereum, and cat-scratch disease. In sarcoidosis, a disease of unknown cause, the granulomas are noncaseating, which may assist in histologic differentiation from tuberculosis.

92. The answer is B (1, 3). *(Robbins, ed 4. pp 876-878.)* Celiac disease, or gluten-sensitive enteropathy, is characterized by malabsorption, abnormal small bowel structure, and intolerance to gluten, a protein found in wheat and rye but not in rice or potatoes. It presents with a typical malabsorption syndrome of weight loss, diarrhea, steatorrhea, bloating, and abnormal absorption tests and is a cause of failure to thrive in children. Celiac disease is associated with increased frequency of HLA-B8 (over 85 percent of cases) and HLA-Dw3 (over 90 percent) antigens, which may indicate a role for immune response genes in pathogenesis. The small bowel mucosa shows villous atrophy with mucosal flattening. Crypts are deepened and show increased mitotic activity, and there is a chronic inflammatory infiltrate in the lamina propria. Immunoperoxidase staining of these inflammatory cells shows large numbers of cells carrying IgA antigliadin antibodies, and a lesser increase in cells carrying IgM antigliadin antibodies. Electron microscopy shows distortion of microvilli, abundant ribonucleoprotein granules, and mitochondria of unusual shape. None of these changes are pathognomonic, however, as they may also be found in tropical sprue and other conditions. With disease lasting 10 years or more there is a 10 to 15 percent chance of developing cancer. Half of these cancers are B-cell lymphomas, and the other half are carcinomas that may arise anywhere in the gastrointestinal tract, but occur especially frequently in the small bowel.

93. The answer is B (1, 3). *(Robbins, ed 4. pp 323-325, 734.)* Epstein-Barr virus (EBV) is contracted by contact with infected saliva, which then enters the epithelial cells of the salivary gland and thereupon enters the B lymphocytes with subsequent viral replication. The viral genome is incorporated into the transformed B lymphocyte DNA. Such transformed lymphocytes are capable of long-term growth in vitro. A virus-related membrane antigen then is found on these transformed B cells that elicits the formation of killer T lymphocytes, which dispose of the latent B cells. Viremia resulting from lysis of B cells is dealt with by virus-neutralizing antibodies that peak 10 to 14 days following infection and are life-long. In Burkitt's lymphoma a suppression or defect in a killer T-cell response to EBV results in a sustained B-cell proliferation, which, if it is persistent, increases the risk for such changes as chromosomal translocations, which may then result in the neoplastic state. This emergence of monoclonal B-cell proliferation from a polyclonal response to the virus may also explain the lymphomas seen in X-linked lymphoproliferative syndrome and in angioimmunoblastic lymphadenopathy.

94. The answer is C (2, 4). *(Robbins, ed 4. pp 301-302.)* The photomicrograph in the question shows an immunoperoxidase reaction, a technique fostered by Sternberger in the early 1970s to identify antigens within cells by the use of an antibody specific for the antigen sought. Following incubation with a specific antibody directed against the target antigen (primary antibody incubation), a secondary antibody incubation is conducted using heterologous immune sera directed against the first antibody. For example, the primary antibody may be rabbit antihuman IgG. If human IgG is present on or within a given cell, binding occurs. Secondary antibody could then be goat antirabbit, which now binds to the rabbit IgG. Then horseradish peroxidase-antiperoxidase conjugate is applied, which links to the antibody complexes. The last step is a chromogen substrate, in this case rust-brown diaminobenzidine. Rust-brown granules indicate a positive reaction. This useful technique (or a modification of it, such as the use of highly specific and sensitive monoclonal antibodies with avidin-biotin conjugate rather than peroxidase-antiperoxidase) is used to identify tumor-associated antigens, viruses and other microorganisms, proteins, and hormones.

95. The answer is E (all). *(Anderson, ed 9. pp 1659-1661.)* Endometrial carcinoma affects menopausal and postmenopausal women, with the peak incidence at 55 to 65 years of age. Although it was much less common than squamous cervical cancer several decades ago, it has not been controlled as effectively as cervical cancer by the Papanicolaou smear technique and therapy, so that it is now more common than invasive cervical cancer. However, the major symptom of endometrial carcinoma, postmenopausal bleeding, results in diagnosis while the tumor is still confined to the uterus (stage I or II), which permits cure by surgery or radiotherapy. The annual death rate in the U.S. from endometrial cancer is 3000, while more than 6000 deaths result from squamous cervical cancer. Risk factors for endometrial cancer include obesity and glucose intolerance or diabetes.

96. The answer is B (1, 3). *(Robbins, ed 4. pp 18-19, 984-987, 1185.)* Necrosis of fat cells occurs in the stromal and peripancreatic fat, in fat depots within the abdominal cavity, and in traumatized breast tissue. Fat necrosis, perhaps the most characteristic histologic change of acute pancreatic necrosis, is thought to take place by the enzymatic hydrolysis of fat, in which one of the end products (fatty acids) is saponified with calcium and deposited as an insoluble granular material. Fat necrosis in traumatized breast tissue is without clinical significance, except that the calcifications may be mistaken for a sign of malignancy during mammographic evaluation.

97. The answer is E (all). *(Robbins, ed 4. pp 1355-1357.)* Diseases that lead to continued tissue synthesis and breakdown may produce hyperuricemia and clinical gout because of the resulting increase in nucleic acid turnover. This form of secondary gout may be seen in polycythemia vera, myeloid metaplasia, chronic leukemia, extensive psoriasis, and sarcoidosis. Cytotoxic drugs used in the chemotherapy of cancer may augment hyperuricemia. Decreased renal excretion of uric acid may also lead to secondary gout. Overproduction of uric acid may result from inborn errors of metabolism, as in the Lesch-Nyhan syndrome (deficiency of the enzyme hypoxanthine-guanine phosphoribosyltransferase (HGPRT).

98. The answer is E (all). *(Anderson, ed 9. pp 757-766.)* In atherosclerosis, primarily a disease of the arterial intima, disintegration of the internal elastic lamina is typical in advanced lesions, and necrosis commonly occurs at the base of the thickened intima. Essential lesions, occurring in the intima, are more numerous in larger than in smaller arteries. Although plaque formations cause little reduction in the size of the lumen of large arteries, atherosclerosis can lead to arterial dilatation and aneurysms.

99. The answer is A (1, 2, 3). *(Robbins, ed 4. pp 151-153.)* Seven well-defined syndromes resulting from genetic defects in enzymes responsible for glycogen metabolism have been described. Six of these diseases, including von Gierke's, Pompe's, and McArdle's, are associated with excess accumulation of glycogen. The seventh disease is characterized by a lack of glycogen. Patients with Tay-Sachs disease have excessive accumulations of a ganglioside.

100. The answer is A (1, 2, 3). *(Robbins, ed 4. pp 1371-1373.)* Granular cell tumors (formerly known as *granular cell myoblastomas*) are benign neoplasms that frequently contain S-100 protein. They originate from Schwann-cell precursors. The most frequent locations are the tongue and subepidermal and subcutaneous tissues of the trunk (breast and many other sites). The eosinophilic cytoplasmic granules are phagolysosomes. These tumors are rarely malignant, though poorly encapsulated, and they frequently cause pseudoepitheliomatous hyperplasia of overlying epithelium, which is difficult to differentiate from squamous cell carcinoma.

101. The answer is A (1, 2, 3). *(Robbins, ed 4. pp 452-455.)* Neurologic dysfunctions are common with deficiencies of the B vitamins pyridoxine, niacin, and riboflavin, which act as coenzymes in cellular oxidative metabolism. Pyridoxine acts as a coenzyme in metabolic functions in the brain, including the synthesis of neurotransmitters. Therefore, B_6 deficiency can result in peripheral neuropathies or birth of retarded infants from pyridoxine-deficient mothers. Niacin deficiency causes degeneration of brain ganglion cells and produces dementia.

102. The answer is C (2, 4). *(Robbins, ed 4. pp 26, 950-953.)* *Hemochromatosis* is a generic term for disorders of iron overload marked by increases in total body iron and deposition of ferritin and hemosiderin in various organs with morphologic and functional damage to those organs. The pathogenesis is not fully understood but involves altered intestinal handling of iron with decreased postabsorption excretion, and alterations in iron metabolism and storage in reticuloendothelial cells. It causes a micronodular pigment cirrhosis with hemosiderin deposition in parenchymal, Kupffer, and bile duct epithelial cells, which is highlighted on Prussian blue staining. Hepatocellular carcinoma is a frequent (15 to 30 percent) complication of pigment cirrhosis. The pancreas shows intense pigmentation with atrophy and loss of parenchymal cells and diffuse interstitial fibrosis. Diabetes is a major feature of the clinical syndrome, but is poorly correlated to the degree of iron deposition in the islets. Other tissues and organs that suffer major deposition of iron include the myocardium, the endocrine glands, skin (melanin and hemosiderin), and testes. Various tests useful in diagnosis reveal increased serum ferritin and plasma iron and decreased iron-binding capacity reflecting increased body iron load. Liver biopsy is definitive when it shows elevated hemosiderin content.

103. The answer is A (1, 2, 3). *(Anderson, ed 9. pp 462, 467-468.)* Eggs of the roundworm *Ascaris* are found in contaminated soil in the southeastern United States. When swallowed, these eggs hatch, reach the small intestinal vessels, and travel to the lungs, where they may produce clinical bronchial asthma and pneumonitis. The New World hookworm, *Necator americanus,* penetrates exposed skin through exposure to larvae-containing soil; these infective filariform larvae reach the pulmonary circulation via the lymphatic and vascular systems and cause alveolar hemorrhages and temporary bronchopneumonia. Rhabditiform *Strongyloides* soil larvae also gain access to the vascular system and pulmonary circuit through penetration of exposed skin and also cause intraalveolar pneumonitis and hemorrhages. *Wuchereria bancrofti* filariae gain access to the human lymphatics (endolymphangitis, elephantiasis) via bites of the *Culex* mosquito; this organism is not noted for producing a pulmonary phase, but it does produce characteristic spermatic cord granulomas.

104. The answer is B (1, 3). *(Robbins, ed 4. pp 61-62, 173-174, 696.)* The electron photomicrograph in the question shows a macrophage, the workhorse of the mononuclear phagocyte system. This wondrous cell is quite possibly the most active cell in the body. It certainly qualifies for the honor if multiple, varied functions are used to judge the competition. A partial list includes endocytosis (phagocytosis of particulate matter including injured cells and bacteria; pinocytosis of molecules in solution), antigen presentation and immunologic trafficking with sensitized T lymphocytes, and lysis of tumor cells. The macrophage also synthesizes and/or elaborates plasminogen activator, elastase, collagenase, some coagulation factors other than factor VIII (such as thromboplastin), neutrophilic chemotactic factor, mediators of inflammation, cyclooxygenase, lipoxygenase glycerol phosphocholine, components of complement, growth factors for wound healing, endogenous pyrogen (interleukin I), and probably other substances. Its internal machinery includes the work of acid hydrolytic enzymes in phagolysosomes. Mast cells and basophils degranulate in anaphylactic reactions. Factor VIII-vWF is a complex of coagulant (factor VIII, made in the liver) and von Willebrand's factor (vWF) that is synthesized in megakaryocytes and vascular endothelium.

105. The answer is B (1, 3). *(Henry, ed 17. pp 655-656, 665-667.)* Since the advent of the Jamshidi biopsy needle in the 1960s and proof that iliac crest marrow accurately reflects the state of the erythron, clinicians have not hesitated in performing or requesting bone marrow examinations of the iliac crest. The procedure's safety records are unquestioned. The practice of using bone marrow biopsy to define and document involvement of bone marrow by both solid and hematopoietic tumors has great value in the staging of patients. Similarly, documenting sideroblastic anemia by demonstrating the presence of ringed sideroblasts in the marrow has great value in clarifying anemias refractory to treatment. However, some clinicians injudiciously order bone marrow examinations in the investigation of iron deficiency anemia to identify stainable iron. In iron deficiency, the serum iron level is low, the iron-binding capacity is high, and the circulating serum transferrin level is high. After treatment with iron, the serum transferrin level will decrease. Evidence for osteoporosis can be established by simple x-rays.

106. The answer is E (all). *(Robbins, ed 4. pp 224-225, 233, 297-299.)* Immunodeficiency states often predispose to the development of neoplasia. The primary immunodeficiencies most clearly associated with an increased incidence of malignancy are common variable immunodeficiency, severe combined immunodeficiency, Wiskott-Aldrich syndrome, and ataxia-telangiectasia (in which defective repair of DNA may also play a role). The neoplasms in these genetic immunodeficiencies are predominantly non-Hodgkin's lymphomas, often immunoblastic, and often extranodal. Secondary immunodeficiency states occur in patients immunosuppressed for organ transplantation and tumors that develop are mainly high-grade, non-Hodgkin's lymphomas, frequently extranodal, especially in the CNS. Transplant patients also show an increased incidence of Kaposi's sarcoma, and a slight increase of squamous cell carcinoma in skin and oral tissues has been reported. The significant increase in neoplasia due to irradiation and radiomimetic drugs—primarily an increase in acute nonlymphoid leukemia—appears to be largely independent of immunosuppression. AIDS, a major devastating example of secondary immunodeficiency, was first recognized in 1981 through the increased incidence of Kaposi's sarcoma in young homosexual men. Subsequent studies established a considerable increase of high-grade, non-Hodgkin's lymphomas in patients infected with human immunodeficiency virus (HIV). Such lymphomas include small noncleaved cell, immunoblastic, and diffuse large cell lymphomas. There also may be an increase in Hodgkin's disease of aggressive type in HIV infection.

107. The answer is D (4). *(Henry, ed 17. p 1130. Morris, N Engl J Med 312:343, 1985.)* The *Vibrio* genus, including *V. cholerae*, is associated with gastrointestinal disease in the Far East, especially India, but is capable of inducing disease in the United States, as in pandemics occurring here around 1832 and in 1849. Along the coasts, especially the northeast and Gulf coasts of the United States, the vibrios increase in numbers in seawater and in seafood and are more likely to cause infections during the late summer and early autumn months. Patients with underlying liver disease, such as alcoholics, and those with immunosuppressive disorders are advised not to ingest raw shellfish during these months because of an increased incidence of disease with the vibrio organisms in these patients. The mycobacteria are acid-fast bacilli associated with tuberculosis and tuberculosis-like diseases; *M. avium-intracellularae* is known to be a frequent organism in AIDS. These organisms are not curved as the vibrios are.

108. The answer is A (1, 2, 3). *(Robbins, ed 4. pp 56-57.)* Leukocytes, including basophils, are involved with the production of derivatives of a very important polyunsaturated fatty acid, arachidonic acid. By a complex two-path cascade system, the metabolites of arachidonic acid eventually yield prostaglandins (vasodilators) and leukotrienes (vasoconstrictors). The biosynthesis begins by activation of cell phospholipase A_2 and C and proceeds either by the action of fatty acid cyclooxygenase on arachidonic acid to form prostaglandins, or by the action of lipoxygenase to yield leukotrienes (hydroperoxyeicosatetraenoic acid in platelets, mast cells, and leukocytes). While many substances can be chemotactic, few are known to be as potent as several of the leukotrienes. Leukotriene B_4 as a chemotactic agent is involved in neutrophil aggregation, while leukotrienes TC_4, TD_4, and TE_4 are involved with increased vascular permeability, bronchoconstriction, and vasoconstriction. Prostaglandin E and prostacyclin probably account for most vasodilatation seen in inflammation. Thus both leukotrienes and prostaglandins contribute to edema. Aspirin and indomethacin can block the actions of cyclooxygenase, thereby inhibiting the biosynthesis of prostaglandin.

109-111. The answers are: 109-B, 110-D, 111-E. *(Robbins, ed 4. pp 294-296, 301-303.)* Acanthosis nigricans is an important skin marker for both benign and malignant conditions. It sometimes results from tumor production of epidermal growth-promoting factors that cause thickening of the stratum spinosum or prickle-cell layer and skin hyperpigmentation of flexures such as axillae and groins. In children it is usually of benign type, but the malignant form of acanthosis nigricans in middle-aged and older persons is often associated (50 percent of cases) with adenocarcinoma. The cancer is most often gastric, but may be lung or uterine. Acanthosis nigricans occurs rarely as a genetic disease. In some of the nongenetic cases there is endocrinopathy, but no cancer is present.

Polycythemia occurring as a paraneoplastic syndrome is usually caused by renal cell carcinoma through production of erythropoietin. The syndrome may also occur with cerebellar hemangioma or hepatocellular carcinoma. Renal cell carcinoma can cause several other paraneoplastic syndromes, including hypercalcemia, Cushing's syndrome, and feminization or masculinization.

A high level of acid phosphatase in the presence of prostatic enlargement is a basis for suspicion of prostatic carcinoma. A normal level is not helpful because only radioimmunoassay procedures are sensitive enough to detect minor elevations.

Unfortunately, levels of serum acid phosphatase are significantly high only when the tumor is advanced. Since total serum acid phosphatase is not specific, it is essential to measure the prostatic fraction, prostatic acid phosphatase, and prostatic-specific antigen, which are more reliable indicators.

Desmin is the intermediate filament specific for tumors showing muscle differentiation, smooth or striated.

Alpha-fetoprotein (AFP), an intrauterine alpha-globulin not normally present in postnatal serum, often shows marked elevation in hepatocellular carcinoma and germ cell tumors of the testis. Benign liver disease (cirrhosis or hepatitis) may cause small-to-moderate elevations. The clinical usefulness of AFP is in following a patient for recurrence of the tumor after therapy, since high levels of serum AFP generally mean recurrence.

112-115. The answers are: 112-B, 113-C, 114-A, 115-D. *(Robbins, ed 4. pp 325, 332, 335, 380-382, 394-396.)* Histoplasma capsulatum causes one of the three major fungal infections in the United States that may result in systemic infection (*Blastomyces* and *Coccidioides* are the other two). Although it commonly produces asymptomatic primary disease, it can result in striking granulomatous inflammation with granulomatous lung disease and possibly sclerosing mediastinitis. Seen most frequently in the Midwest, and inhaled from contaminated soil, it forms a yeast-like pathogenic phase in the host and may cause acute, chronic progressive, or asymptomatic disease, the last being the most common outcome.

Lepromatous leprosy may result in a leonine facies, as does onchocerciasis and leishmaniasis, because of thickened, overhanging facial folds. In the United States, leprosy is found primarily in Florida, California, Texas, Louisiana, and Hawaii. The Fite stain (fuchsin and formalin) is the usual acid-fast stain for *Mycobacterium leprae* and produces blue bacteria.

Rocky Mountain spotted fever is transmitted to man by ticks, as is Lyme disease. Rocky Mountain spotted fever—an acute infectious disease caused by *Rickettsia rickettsii* and characterized by muscle pain, high fever, and skin eruptions—is endemic throughout North America. Rickettsiae typically invade the walls of blood vessels with resultant hemorrhage and thrombosis.

Yellow fever is an acute infectious disease of variable severity and short duration. It is an arthropod-borne (*Aedes* mosquito), hemorrhagic disease of subtropical and tropical New World areas, caused by a single-stranded RNA togavirus. It results in hepatocellular damage with jaundice and hematemesis.

Gram-negative bacteria have cell walls containing endotoxins (lipopolysaccharide-protein complexes) that are released from disintegrating bacteria to cause such effects of gram-negative sepsis as fever, increased capillary permeability with shock, and disseminated intravascular coagulation.

116-119. The answers are: 116-C, 117-D, 118-E, 119-B. *(Robbins, ed 4. pp 1453, 1454, 1460, 1461.)* Long-standing diabetes mellitus is a major cause of blindness in the United States and Europe (25 percent of cases of acquired blindness in the U.S.). Diabetic retinopathy is the most common form, but cataracts and glaucoma occur also. Two major types of diabetic retinopathy, nonproliferative and proliferative, exist with the former characterized by microaneurysms, hemorrhages, and thickened retinal capillaries (microangiopathy). In proliferative retinopathy, new capillary formation and fibrosis eventually lead to blindness or decreased visual acuity.

Keratomalacia, which is due to severe, protracted vitamin A deficiency, is a major problem in Southeast Asia, Africa, and Central and South America, where it causes blindness in about one quarter million children annually. Dryness, softening, and destruction of the cornea occur, while characteristic eye changes include Bitot's spots—a localized form of keratomalacia with small gray plaques representing thickened, keratinized epithelium.

Trachoma, a common cause of blindness in hot, arid regions of the Third World, is caused by *Chlamydia trachomatis*, serotypes A to C. Conjunctival infection is followed by lymphoid follicular hyperplasia and, subsequently, pannus invades the cornea and leads to blindness.

Retinitis pigmentosa is a rare degeneration of the retinal outer receptor layer and underlying pigment epithelium; it is inherited as an autosomal dominant, or recessive, or sex-linked recessive trait. Losses of night vision and, eventually, central vision are prominent.

Silver-wire arterioles are seen in severe arteriosclerotic retinopathy when sclerotic opacity obscures intravascular blood completely.

120-123. The answers are: 120-C, 121-E, 122-A, 123-D. *(Robbins, ed 4. pp 173-180, 743-744, 1040-1041, 1044.)* All five immunoglobulins are polypeptides with two light and two heavy chains linked by disulfide bonds. The Ig molecule consists of two fragments of Fab, which are capable of binding antigen, and one Fc fragment. Light chains are of two types, kappa and lambda. Heavy chains are of five major types forming five distinct immunoglobulin classes on the basis of the heavy chains that account for the antigenic differences.

IgA is synthesized by mucosal plasma cells of the GI tract, lung, and urinary tract—thus making it the immunoglobulin of "secretory immunity"—and is found in saliva, sweat, nasal secretion, and tears. It is secreted as dimer bound to a secretory piece that stabilizes the molecule against proteolysis. In IgA nephropathy (Berger's disease), circulating IgA immune complex is present in 50 percent of patients and a diffuse renal mesangial proliferation with IgA deposition occurs.

Local anaphylactic reactions include hay fever, bronchial asthma, certain food allergies, and urticarial reactions to drugs or injected antigens. Systemic anaphylaxis may result from injection of antisera or penicillin and may cause severe shock or death. Type I hypersensitivity (anaphylaxis) occurs when exposure to antigen leads to production of cytotropic IgE antibodies that become fixed by their Fc portions to mast cells and basophils. On reexposure, antigen combines with the cell-bound antibody and this is followed by mast cell degranulation with discharge of primary mediators (histamine). Secondary mediators (leukotrienes, prostaglandin) are released via cell membrane phospholipids.

IgM is the first immunoglobulin to respond to an antigenic stimulus and is the largest Ig. Waldenström's macroglobulinemia is a plasma cell dyscrasia characterized by infiltration of bone marrow, lymph nodes, liver, and spleen by neoplastic B cells that secrete a monoclonal IgM immunoglobulin, leading to macroglobulinemia. Serum electrophoresis shows an M-protein spike and diagnosis rests on the typical bone marrow findings and the M-protein spike due to IgM in the serum.

Most of the circulating human gamma globulin (80 percent) is of the IgG class. It crosses the placenta and is the major protective immunoglobulin in the neonate. IgG has Fc receptors and activates complement.

Hematology

DIRECTIONS: Each question below contains five suggested responses. Select the **one best** response to each question.

124. The photomicrograph below was taken from a soft tissue swelling in the cheek and mandible of a 17-year-old female patient. The cytoplasmic vacuoles would react with which one of the following?

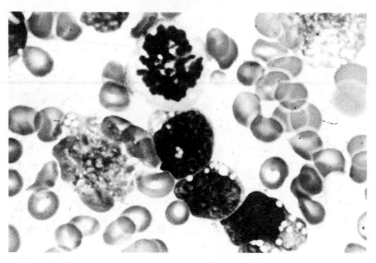

(A) Myeloperoxidase
(B) Oil red O
(C) Nonspecific esterase
(D) Chloracetate esterase
(E) Periodic acid–Schiff (PAS)

125. The neutrophil in the photomicrograph shown below was obtained from peripheral blood and is most likely to be found in association with

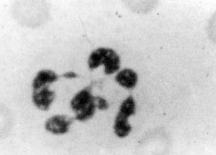

(A) folic acid deficiency
(B) infection
(C) iron deficiency
(D) malignancy
(E) ingestion of a marrow-toxic agent

126. The graph below depicts the results of a red cell osmotic fragility test. The broken-line curve represents which of the following?

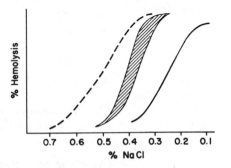

(A) Glucose 6-phosphate dehydrogenase deficiency
(B) Thalassemia
(C) Hereditary spherocytosis
(D) Drug-induced hemolytic anemia
(E) Normal response

127. In the photomicrograph below, the nucleated cell that is located next to the neutrophil has a gray-pink cytoplasm and is

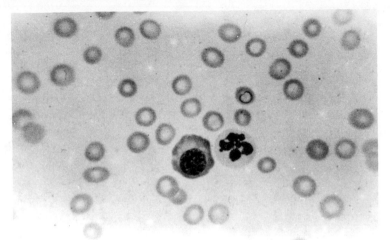

(A) a polychromatophilic megaloblast
(B) a plasma cell
(C) an orthochromatic normoblast
(D) a myelocyte
(E) a myeloblast

128. Which of the following laboratory findings is LEAST likely to be present in a patient with sickle cell anemia?

(A) Normochromic anemia
(B) Increased number of target cells
(C) Elevated reticulocyte count
(D) Elevated erythrocyte sedimentation rate
(E) Increased hemoglobin F

129. Patients with sickle cell trait have which of the following genotypes?

(A) $\alpha^s \alpha \beta \beta$
(B) $\alpha^s \alpha^s \beta \beta$
(C) $\alpha \alpha \beta \beta^s$
(D) $\alpha \alpha \beta^s \beta^s$
(E) $\alpha \alpha^s \beta \beta^s$

130. The causes of secondary aplastic anemia include all the following EXCEPT

(A) whole body irradiation
(B) alkylating agents
(C) chloramphenicol
(D) myelophthisic anemia
(E) viral hepatitis

131. Vitamin K is required for the synthesis of all the following EXCEPT

(A) prothrombin
(B) clotting factor VII
(C) clotting factor VIII
(D) clotting factor IX
(E) clotting factor X

132. Which of the following substances inhibits platelet aggregation?

(A) Prostacyclin (PGI₂)
(B) Epinephrine
(C) Adenosine diphosphate
(D) 5-Hydroxytryptamine
(E) Thrombin

133. The photomicrograph below is of peripheral blood from a patient with splenomegaly, anemia, and pancytopenia. If hairy cell leukemia is suspected, which of the following would be useful in establishing the diagnosis?

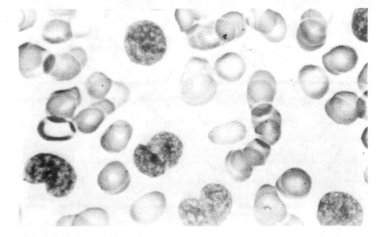

(A) Myeloperoxidase stain
(B) Sudan black B
(C) Acid phosphatase stain
(D) Leukocyte alkaline phosphatase
(E) Nonspecific esterase

134. The photomicrograph below is of the spleen from an adult patient who had marked splenomegaly. Which of the following abnormalities is most compatible with the changes seen in the spleen?

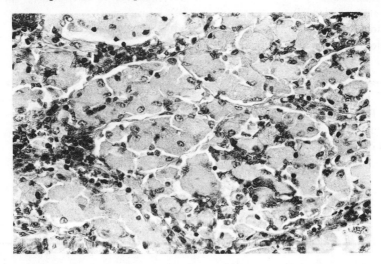

(A) Reduced levels of glucocerebrosidase activity
(B) Glucose 6-phosphate dehydrogenase deficiency
(C) Glucuronidase deficiency
(D) Lysosomal glucosidase deficiency
(E) Trihexosylceramide α-galactosidase deficiency

135. Acute idiopathic thrombocytopenic purpura (ITP) in children is characterized by

(A) an insidious onset
(B) being more common in females
(C) a history of recent viral infection
(D) megakaryocytic hypoplasia
(E) a high mortality

136. An 11-year-old Jamaican boy develops a massive benign enlargement of the cervical lymph nodes associated with fever and leukocytosis. Which of the following lymph node disorders could account for these findings?

(A) Toxoplasmosis
(B) Histiocytic medullary reticulosis
(C) Burkitt's disease
(D) Sinus histiocytosis with massive lymphadenopathy (SHML)
(E) Angioimmunoblastic lymphadenopathy with dysproteinemia

137. The photomicrograph below was taken after 30 minutes of incubation at 37°C of a mixture of one drop of blood and two drops of an aqueous 2% sodium metabisulfite solution. The appearance of the erythrocytes in this preparation shows that they contain

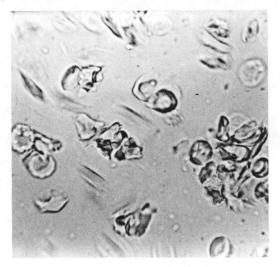

(A) hemoglobin A
(B) hemoglobin A$_2$
(C) hemoglobin C
(D) hemoglobin F
(E) hemoglobin S

138. The photomicrograph below is from the bone marrow of a patient with weakness. All the following may be associated with this abnormality EXCEPT

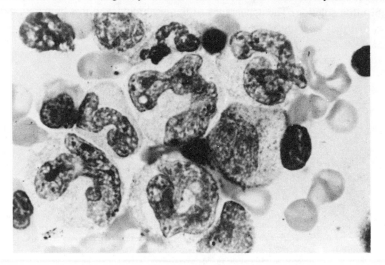

(A) pernicious anemia
(B) hyperthyroidism
(C) celiac disease
(D) HTLV
(E) alcoholism

139. The cells shown in the photomicrograph below are usually increased in the peripheral blood in all the following EXCEPT

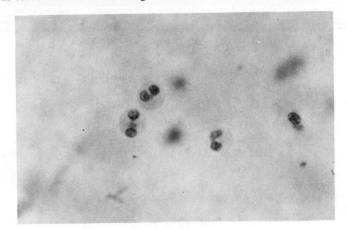

(A) eczema and pemphigus
(B) bronchial asthma
(C) some cases of Hodgkin's disease
(D) adrenocortical stimulation
(E) parasitic infections

140. A bone marrow aspirate was obtained from a 70-year-old man whose symptoms included weakness, weight loss, and recurrent infections. Laboratory findings included proteinuria, anemia, and an abnormal component in serum proteins. A photomicrograph of the bone marrow aspirate is shown below. The most probable diagnosis is

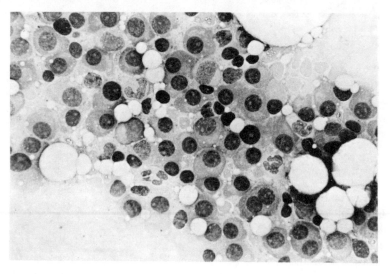

(A) monomyelocytic leukemia
(B) histiocytic leukemia
(C) multiple myeloma
(D) Gaucher's disease
(E) leukemic reticuloendotheliosis

141. Typical findings in a patient with von Willebrand's disease include all the following EXCEPT

(A) decreased levels of factor VIII
(B) decreased glass bead adhesion of platelets
(C) prolonged bleeding time
(D) frequent hemarthrosis and spontaneous joint hemorrhage
(E) menorrhagia

142. δ-Aminolevulinic acid is excreted in increased amounts in the urine of patients with

(A) lead poisoning
(B) carcinoma of the pancreas
(C) chronic pyelonephritis
(D) vitamin C intoxication
(E) ulcerative colitis

Questions 143-144

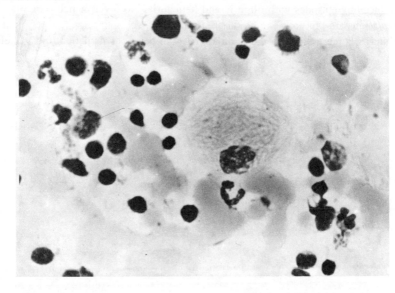

143. The cell in the photomicrograph above was found in a bone marrow aspirate from a 25-year-old man. Such a cell is generally considered pathognomonic for

(A) Niemann-Pick disease
(B) histiocytic lymphoma
(C) megaloblastic anemia
(D) Gaucher's disease
(E) myelogenous leukemia

144. All the following statements concerning the disease associated with the cell shown above are true EXCEPT

(A) the pathognomonic cells are typically 20 to 100 μm in diameter and have a wrinkled, striated cytoplasm
(B) inheritance is autosomal dominant with variable penetrance
(C) the serum level of acid phosphatase is frequently elevated
(D) an excess amount of sphingolipid is stored in body tissues
(E) three types of the disease can be differentiated genetically and clinically

145. A woman who is 5 weeks post partum (normal delivery, healthy child) develops bleeding episodes with oliguria and hematuria. No fever or neurologic manifestations are present. The blood urea nitrogen level is 65 mg/dl; a peripheral blood smear is represented in the photomicrograph below. This patient most likely has

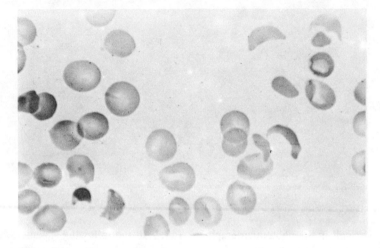

(A) thrombotic thrombocytopenic purpura
(B) autoimmune thrombocytopenic purpura
(C) hemolytic uremic syndrome
(D) disseminated intravascular coagulopathy
(E) sickle cell crisis

---

146. All the following are known to cause splenomegaly EXCEPT

(A) sickle cell disease
(B) Hodgkin's disease
(C) chronic lymphocytic leukemia (CLL)
(D) hairy cell leukemia
(E) polycythemia vera

147. Non-Hodgkin's lymphomas (NHLs) that exhibit a nodular growth pattern may be characterized by which of the following?

(A) Increased frequency in adolescents
(B) Predominant T cell type
(C) Better prognosis than in the diffuse type
(D) Predominance in males
(E) Well-differentiated lymphocytic lymphoma

148. A 38-year-old man presents with a red, maculopapular rash, Coombs' positive hemolytic anemia, generalized lymphadenopathy, splenomegaly, hepatomegaly, fever, fatigue, and weight loss. The lymph node biopsy specimen seen in the photomicrograph below shows effacement and vascular proliferation. This constellation points to a diagnosis of

(A) lymphopathia venereum
(B) immunoblastic lymphadenopathy
(C) mucocutaneous lymph node syndrome
(D) acute leukemia
(E) malignant histiocytosis

149. The cells seen in the photomicrograph below were removed from a patient suffering from anemia and stained with an iron stain. This patient is most likely to have

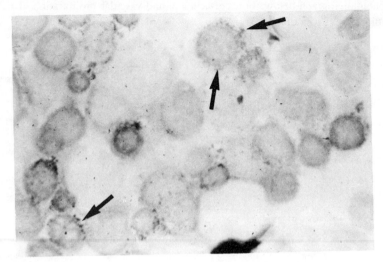

(A) iron deficiency anemia
(B) acute blood loss
(C) B_{12} deficiency
(D) B_2 deficiency
(E) pyridoxine deficiency

150. The presence in serum of a mu heavy-chain protein is a distinctive feature of which of the following diseases?

(A) Chronic lymphocytic leukemia
(B) Macroglobulinemia
(C) Lymphocytic lymphoma
(D) Plasma cell myeloma
(E) Multiple myeloma

151. The bone marrow biopsy shown below was performed because of spleno-megaly and anemia in an adult. On the basis of the appearance of the bone mar-row core, choose the most likely diagnosis.

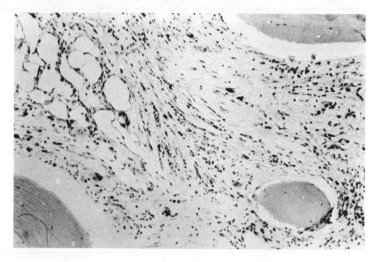

(A) Chronic myeloid leukemia (CML)
(B) Aplastic anemia
(C) Acute leukemia
(D) Myeloid metaplasia with myelofibrosis
(E) Microangiopathic hemolytic anemia

152. A 20-year-old man presents in the emergency room with a lymphoma involving the mediastinum that is pro-ducing respiratory distress. The lym-phocytes are most likely to have cell surface markers characteristic of which of the following?

(A) B cells
(B) T cells
(C) Macrophages
(D) Dendritic reticulum cells
(E) Langerhans cells

153. Transferrin shows all the follow-ing characteristics EXCEPT

(A) normally about 33 percent satura-tion with iron
(B) increased saturation in hemochro-matosis
(C) increased saturation in severe liver disease
(D) decreased saturation in marrow hypoplasia
(E) decreased saturation in iron defi-ciency anemia

154. An elderly woman enters the hospital with an abdominal mass, anemia, and weakness. At surgery, an infiltrating retroperitoneal mass is found involving the mesenteric lymph nodes and right kidney. A biopsy specimen from one of the lymph nodes is shown and is compatible with large-cell immunoblastic lymphoma. This neoplasm is associated with all the following EXCEPT

(A) predominant B-cell origin
(B) prior immunologic disorder
(C) early dissemination to bone marrow
(D) rapid death if untreated
(E) plasmacytoid or polymorphous features

155. An anemic patient has the following red cell indexes: mean corpuscular volume, 70 μm^3 (normal: 90 ± 7); mean corpuscular hemoglobin, 22 g/100 ml (normal: 29 ± 2); and mean corpuscular hemoglobin concentration, 34 percent (normal: 34 ± 2). These values are most consistent with a diagnosis of

(A) folic acid deficiency anemia
(B) iron deficiency anemia
(C) pernicious anemia
(D) thalassemia minor
(E) sideroblastic anemia

156. Chronic myeloid leukemia is LEAST likely to be associated with

(A) splenomegaly
(B) basophilia
(C) translocation t (8; 14)
(D) thrombocytosis
(E) low leukocyte alkaline phosphatase

157. During the induction of an immune response, which cell is thought to process the initiating antigen?

(A) Eosinophil
(B) Basophil
(C) Macrophage
(D) T cell
(E) B cell

158. A young child has recurrent bacterial infections, eczema, thrombocytopenia, lymphadenopathy, and the absence of delayed-type hypersensitivity. The most likely diagnosis is

(A) Pelger-Huët anomaly
(B) Wiskott-Aldrich syndrome
(C) Chédiak-Higashi syndrome
(D) chronic granulomatous disease of childhood
(E) nodular-sclerosing Hodgkin's disease

159. A 25-year-old woman with known systemic lupus erythematosus presents with jaundice, splenomegaly, peripheral blood schistocytes, and a reticulocyte count of 24 percent. The antibody most likely to be responsible for this complex reacts in vitro at

(A) 5°C
(B) 20°C
(C) 25°C
(D) 37°C
(E) 56°C

DIRECTIONS: Each question below contains four suggested responses of which **one or more** is correct. Select

A	if	**1, 2, and 3**	are correct
B	if	**1 and 3**	are correct
C	if	**2 and 4**	are correct
D	if	**4**	is correct
E	if	**1, 2, 3, and 4**	are correct

160. The binucleated or bilobed tumor giant cell with prominent acidophilic "owl-eye" nucleoli shown in the photomicrograph below

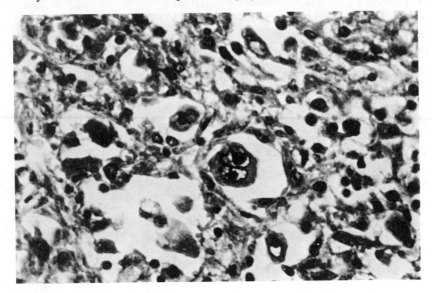

(1) is necessary but not sufficient for the diagnosis of Hodgkin's disease
(2) is sometimes referred to as the "lacunar cell"
(3) may be seen in benign conditions
(4) is a rapidly proliferating tumor cell seen in middivision

Questions 161-163

In the photomicrograph shown below, cells aspirated from bone marrow show megaloblastic erythroid changes.

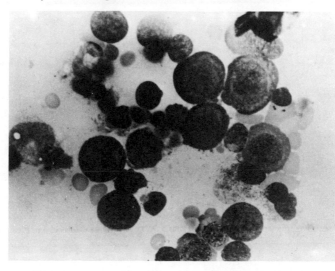

161. The cytologic features in *peripheral* blood that would be consistent with the megaloblastic bone marrow aspirate shown in the photomicrograph include

(1) macrocytes with mean corpuscular volumes exceeding 110 μm^3
(2) numerous myeloblasts
(3) neutrophils with more than the usual three to four segments
(4) secondary polycythemia

162. The megaloblasts shown could be found in bone marrow aspirates from patients who have

(1) erythroleukemia
(2) severe folate and B_{12} deficiency
(3) a history of treatment with anti-folates for leukemia
(4) vitamin A–responsive anemia

163. This bone marrow aspirate is an example of megaloblastic erythroid changes and reveals

(1) a decreased myeloid to erythroid ratio (1:1)
(2) giant band forms with maturation arrested in the granulocytic series
(3) increased mitotic figures in red cell precursors
(4) megaloblastic platelet precursors

Questions 164-166

The amorphous material deposited in the section of tongue below stains pink with Congo red stain and in polarized light appears apple-green in color.

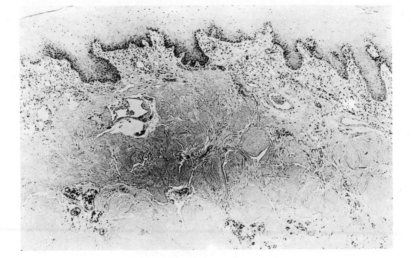

164. Dependable laboratory studies that would aid in the diagnosis of this process include

(1) serum electrophoresis
(2) rectal biopsy or biopsy of clinically abnormal joint synovium
(3) increased absorption of Congo red and Evans blue dyes from the circulation
(4) immunoelectrophoresis on concentrated urine samples

165. Clinical features associated with primary distribution of this material include

(1) diarrhea and malabsorption
(2) cardiac failure unresponsive to digitalis administration
(3) polyarthritis with thickening of periarticular tissues
(4) peripheral neuropathy

166. The presence of this material in an elderly man who has macroglossia and atypical marrow plasmacytosis would be

(1) expected because it occurs frequently in the geriatric population
(2) associated with the presence of M-type serum proteins or Bence Jones proteinuria
(3) almost invariably associated with an increased concentration of normal immunoglobulins
(4) associated with depositions of similar amorphous material in the heart, ligaments, skin, and peripheral nerves

167. Mechanisms that contribute to the decreased erythrocyte survival in autoimmune hemolytic anemia include which of the following?

(1) Complement-mediated lysis
(2) Decreased hemoglobin synthesis
(3) Increased phagocytosis of erythrocytes by the reticuloendothelial system
(4) Hemosiderin deposition

168. A 21-year-old man being discussed at a tumor board has been determined to have Hodgkin's disease and lymphocyte predominance and is thought to be in clinical stage IIA. Statements that apply to his case include which of the following?

(1) There are few Reed-Sternberg cells in the biopsies
(2) He may have fever, pruritus, and weight loss
(3) The involved lymph nodes are on the same side of the diaphragm
(4) The prognosis is fair to good

169. Clinical and laboratory features of paroxysmal nocturnal hemoglobinuria (PNH) include

(1) hemosiderinuria
(2) venous thromboses
(3) positive acid-serum lysis
(4) prior aplastic anemia

DIRECTIONS: The group of questions below consists of lettered headings followed by a set of numbered items. For each numbered item select the **one** lettered heading with which it is **most** closely associated. Each lettered heading may be used **once, more than once, or not at all.**

Questions 170-174

For each description below, choose the type of leukemia with which it is most likely to be associated.

(A) Acute lymphoblastic leukemia
(B) Acute myeloblastic leukemia (M1)
(C) Acute promyelocytic leukemia (M3)
(D) Chronic lymphocytic leukemia
(E) Hairy cell leukemia

170. Auer rods are frequently present in the leukemic cells

171. It is associated with a short course and diffuse intravascular coagulation

172. It occurs in older adults, produces relatively few symptoms, and is associated with the longest survival

173. The enzyme TdT is often present in leukemic cells; lymphadenopathy is characteristic and striking

174. It constitutes about 20 percent of childhood leukemias and relapse is common following chemotherapy in older adults

Hematology
Answers

124. The answer is B. *(Henry, ed 17. pp 721, 737-738. Robbins, ed 4. pp 715-716.)* Burkitt's lymphoma, or undifferentiated lymphoma, is characterized by a rapid proliferation of primitive lymphoid cells with thick nuclear membranes, multiple nucleoli, and intensely basophilic cytoplasm when stained with Wright's stain. The cells are often mixed with macrophages in biopsy, giving a starry-sky appearance. The vacuoles contain lipid and this would be reflected by a positive oil-red-O reaction. PAS stain is nonspecific but does mark neutrophils and acute lymphoblastic leukemia cells. Nonspecific esterase is found predominantly within monocytes but also in megakaryocytes and to a minor extent in myelomonocytes. Chloracetate esterase and myeloperoxidase are primarily found within the lysosomes of granulocytes, including neutrophils, promyelocytes, and faintly in rare monocytes.

125. The answer is A. *(Wintrobe, ed 8. pp 572-573.)* In contrast to a normal, mature neutrophil, which has from two to five nuclear lobes, the neutrophil shown has at least six lobes and is an illustration of neutrophilic hypersegmentation. Granulocytic hypersegmentation is significant and among the first hematologic findings in the peripheral blood of patients who have megaloblastic anemia in its developmental stages. Neutrophilic hypersegmentation is generally considered a sensitive indicator of megaloblastic anemia, which can be caused by a deficiency either in vitamin B_{12}, in folate, or in both.

126. The answer is C. *(Henry, ed 17. pp 671-673. Robbins, ed 4. pp 663-665.)* Spherocytes in a peripheral blood smear show a smaller diameter than normal and an apparent increase in hemoglobin concentration because of a decrease in cell surface, with consequent deeper staining for hemoglobin. Spectrin lacks the ability to bind protein 4.1 in this autosomal dominant disorder, yielding a skeleton defect of the red cell membrane. Other proteins that help maintain the shape of the red cell include protein 3 and ankyrin, which bridges the spectrin and the cell membrane protein 3. The disorder can be diagnosed in the laboratory by the osmotic fragility test (which the graph shows, with the shaded area reflecting a normal response to a hypotonic solution). Spherocytes will lyse at a higher concentration of sodium chloride than will normal red cells. Flat hypochromic cells, as those in thalassemia, have a greater capacity to expand in dilute salt solution and thus lyse at a lower concentration (which is seen in the unbroken curve to the far right). The longer the incu-

81

bation of the red cells in these salt concentrations, the greater the response to osmotic change.

127. The answer is A. *(Williams, ed 4. pp 453-454.)* The cell in question is much larger than the other red cells and has an immature nucleus with coarse, clumped chromatin. These features help to identify it as a nucleated red cell exhibiting megaloblastic maturation. The cell might be confused with a plasma cell, but plasma cells exhibit clumped chromatin that stains a dark purple, a deep blue cytoplasm, and nuclei that are small and eccentric and often lie next to perinuclear clear zones.

128. The answer is D. *(Braunwald, ed 11. pp 1520-1523. Henry, ed 17. pp 679-680.)* Blood from patients who have sickle cell anemia exhibits a low erythrocyte sedimentation rate (ESR). The irregular shape of sickle cells prevents the rouleaux formation that is prerequisite for a normal ESR. Sickle cell anemia is classified as a normocytic, normochromic, and hemolytic anemia in which target cells, found in increased numbers, can compose up to 30 percent of peripheral blood cells, and in which reticulocytosis—as a reflection of an increased rate of erythropoiesis in the hyperplastic bone marrow—is persistently 10 percent above normal. In addition, electrophoretic findings reveal an elevation of hemoglobin F up to 40 percent, the presence of hemoglobin S in a range of 60 to 99 percent, and the absence of hemoglobin A.

129. The answer is C. *(Robbins, ed 4. pp 666-668.)* The abnormal chain in sickle cell hemoglobin is the beta chain and is designated β^s. The alpha chains are normal in both sickle cell disease and trait; an α^s allele does not exist. Persons with a normal adult hemoglobin would be $\alpha\alpha\beta\beta$; those with sickle cell disease would be $\alpha\alpha\beta^s\beta^s$; therefore, persons with sickle trait would be $\alpha\alpha\beta\beta^s$. Some people may inherit more than one genetic mutation and thus produce not only hemoglobin S but hemoglobin C or D or another abnormal hemoglobin. The genotype for these people would be written to reflect such combined defects.

130. The answer is D. *(Robbins, ed 4. pp 688-690.)* Hematopoietic stem cell failure occurs in aplastic anemia, probably because of defective stem cells or their immunologic suppression. Pancytopenia results, although selective suppression with pure red cell aplasia, agranulocytosis, or thrombocytopenia may occur. In 50 percent of cases, aplastic anemia is idiopathic or primary, but there are many physical and chemical causes of secondary aplastic anemia. Whole body irradiation is the major physical cause. Chemical causes include many drugs, such as alkylating agents, antimetabolites, and the antibiotic chloramphenicol. Severe aplastic anemia may occur following viral hepatitis of the non-A, non-B type, or following infectious mononucleosis. In myelophthisic anemia, marrow failure is due to marrow replacement by metastatic tumor or other lesions, but no association with stem cell defects exists.

131. The answer is C. *(Williams, ed 4. pp 1285-1286. Wintrobe, ed 8. p 410.)* Vitamin K is not required for the biosynthesis of coagulation factor VIII, which has an uncertain participation as a trace protein in the intrinsic coagulation pathway and is also known as the antihemophilic factor. Vitamin K, although its biochemical mode of action remains unclear, is required for the biosynthesis and maintenance of normal concentrations of coagulation factors II (prothrombin), VII, IX, and X.

132. The answer is A. *(Robbins, ed 4. pp 95-97.)* Prostacyclin inhibits platelet aggregation, probably by increasing cyclic AMP levels within the platelets, whereas all the other agents listed promote it. Other potent inhibitors of platelet aggregation include mercurials and chemicals that react with sulfhydryl groups.

133. The answer is C. *(Williams, ed 4. pp 1025-1028. Wintrobe, ed 8. pp 1715-1718.)* Since 1966, hairy cell leukemia has been diagnosed with increasing frequency. This specialized form of leukemia should be suspected in patients with splenomegaly; pancytopenia, including thrombocytopenia; bleeding; fatigue; and leukemic lymphocyte-like cells in the peripheral blood demonstrating cytoplasmic projections at the cell periphery ("hairy" cells). These cells stain for acid phosphatase, and the reaction is refractory to treatment with tartaric acid (tartrate-resistant acid phosphatase, or TRAP).

134. The answer is A. *(Robbins, ed 4. pp 146-154.)* The photomicrograph in the question shows the presence of lipid-laden macrophages replacing much of the splenic parenchyma. The macrophages have a somewhat vacuolated cytoplasm, which is characteristic of Gaucher's disease. This is an autosomal recessive disease characterized by a reduction or a deficiency of glucocerebrosidase. Thus glucocerebroside accumulates mainly in the mononuclear phagocytic system. Three clinical types occur. The classic is type I, which occurs in adults and generally spares the central nervous system with the glucocerebrosides limited to the mononuclear phagocyte system of the spleen, liver, and bone marrow. This is mainly found in European Jewish patients and is the most common form of Gaucher's disease. Type II is the infantile form, which involves the brain and presents no detectable glucocerebrosidase activity. Death occurs at an early age. Type III may be thought of as being an intermediate between types I and II; it is found in adolescent patients and mainly involves the mononuclear phagocyte system early but will involve the brain by the third decade of life. Trihexosylceramide α-galactosidase deficiency is Fabry's disease, which is characterized by angiokeratomas of the skin resulting in marked ceramide trihexoside accumulations within the endothelial and smooth muscle cells of blood vessels, ganglion cells, heart, renal tubules, and glomeruli. Glucosidase deficiency is type II glycogen storage disease, which is one of the variants of liver phosphorylase deficiency. Glucose 6-phosphate dehydrogenase deficiency results in hemolytic disease in both sexes, with the male more severely affected.

135. The answer is C. *(Robbins, ed 4. pp 692-695.)* In acute idiopathic thrombocytopenic purpura (ITP), which occurs predominantly in children under 8 years of age, there is an acute onset about 2 weeks after a viral infection (rubella, viral hepatitis, infectious mononucleosis). There is no female predominance as seen in chronic ITP, which is most frequent in females 20 to 50 years old and is characterized by an insidious onset. Both acute and chronic forms are associated with increased platelet destruction and normal or increased megakaryocytes in bone marrow. Most patients with acute ITP make a spontaneous recovery, although cerebral hemorrhage may occur and accounts for most of the few deaths.

136. The answer is D. *(Anderson, ed 9. pp 1436, 1440-1442.)* Clinicians and pathologists alike should be familiar with the benign syndrome of lymph node enlargement called *sinus histiocytosis with massive lymphadenopathy*. This is a self-limiting, invariably benign disorder found classically in young, black, African and Caribbean patients, but it has been found in others as well. It is characterized clinically by profound enlargement of regional cervical lymph nodes, fever, and leukocytosis. Histologically, the lymph nodes show marked histiocytic proliferation within the sinuses, with engulfment of lymphocytes within the histiocytes. There may be skin involvement, and histiocytes containing phagocytosed lymphocytes may be present in the skin biopsy specimen. The patients predictably revert to normal within a period of months. Histiocytic medullary reticulosis is a disease in which a form of malignant histiocytes is found in lymph node sinuses, with engulfed red cells found within the neoplastic histiocytes (erythrophagocytosis). Primitive, round lymphoblastic tumor cells are found in tissue taken from patients with Burkitt's lymphoma.

137. The answer is E. *(Henry, ed 17. p 679.)* The photomicrograph shown in the question demonstrates the results of the metabisulfite sickling test for detecting the presence of hemoglobin S. The test does not differentiate homozygous from heterozygous states. Red cells that contain large amounts of normal or abnormal hemoglobins other than S rarely exhibit sickling. The test is based on the fact that erythrocytes containing a large proportion of hemoglobin S sickle in solutions of low oxygen content. Metabisulfite is a reducing substance that enhances the process of deoxygenation.

138. The answer is D. *(Robbins, ed 4. pp 679-685.)* The photomicrograph in the question shows the presence of megaloblasts accompanied by unusually large neutrophils and precursors. These abnormalities may be caused by either a deficiency or lack of absorption of vitamin B_{12} or of folic acid. In addition to diets deficient in these two substances, any condition leading to poor absorption of them will also lead to megaloblastic anemia. Thus malabsorption (as in celiac disease), gastrectomy, infiltrative disorders of the bowel (including lymphoma and collagen vascular disease such as scleroderma), infections by the fish tapeworm, and metabolic disorders (such as hyperthyroidism and increased demand for folic acid as in advanced stages of malignancy) all will lead to reduced levels of vitamin B_{12} and folic acid. A deficiency of either vitamin B_{12} or folic acid will lead to maturational arrest of the red cell precursors, which yields large and apparently immature red cell precursors—hence the name *megaloblastic*. The nuclei of red cell precursors are in an immature stage for the maturation of the cytoplasm, which results in an unusually large nucleus. Deficiency in vitamin B_{12} and folic acid leads to abnormalities or inadequate synthesis of DNA, which results in a delayed or blocked mitotic division. There is no abnormality in the synthesis of RNA or cytoplasmic protein, and that portion of the cell continues to mature.

139. The answer is D. *(Braunwald, ed 11. pp 282-283.)* The cells shown are eosinophils, and eosinophilic leukocytosis (eosinophilia) is defined as an absolute count exceeding $500/mm^3$. Causes include cutaneous allergic reactions, allergic disorders such as asthma or hay fever, Hodgkin's disease, and parasitic infections (trichinosis, schistosomiasis, strongyloidiasis). Adrenocortical stimulation by administration of corticosteroids may cause eosinophilic leukopenia (eosinopenia), but not eosinophilia. The most common cause of eosinophilia is probably allergy to drugs such as iodides, aspirin, and sulfonamides; eosinophilia is also seen in collagen vascular diseases (rheumatoid arthritis, allergic angiitis). Marked eosinophilia occurs in hypereosinophilic syndromes including Loeffler's syndrome and idiopathic hypereosinophilic syndrome ($50,000$ to $100,000$ eosinophils/mm^3). Corticosteroid therapy induces remission.

140. The answer is C. *(Wintrobe, ed 8. pp 1744-1748.)* The bone marrow aspirate exhibits a proliferation of plasma cells that are characterized by well-defined perinuclear clear zones and by dense cytoplasmic basophilia due to increased RNA accumulations. Weakness, weight loss, recurrent infections, proteinuria, anemia, and abnormal proliferation of plasma cells in the bone marrow are findings that highly suggest the presence of multiple myeloma, a plasma cell dyscrasia. The more definitive diagnostic criteria are findings of M-component in the results of serum electrophoresis and plasma cell levels above 15 percent in the bone marrow. Multiple myeloma, occurring more commonly in males than in females, shows an increasing incidence with increasing age, and most patients are in their seventies.

141. The answer is D. *(Williams, ed 4. p 1498.)* Hemarthroses do not occur frequently in patients who have von Willebrand's disease and usually are caused by trauma. A prolonged bleeding time affects most of the patients and, together with a moderate deficiency in coagulation factor VIII, is usually acceptable for establishing the diagnosis of von Willebrand's disease. Decreased retention of platelets in glass bead filters, normal numbers of platelets, and menorrhagia are usual findings, but petechiae rarely occur. The most common symptoms include epistaxis and increased susceptibility to bruises.

142. The answer is A. *(Robbins, ed 4. pp 492-494.)* Increased amounts of δ-aminolevulinic acid (ALA) and coproporphyrin are found in the urine of patients who have ingested lead. Lead interferes with erythropoiesis by inhibiting the activity of several enzymes, including δ-ALA synthetase and ALA dehydrase. Thus the various degrees of anemia that are usually associated with lead poisoning are more likely to be mediated by interference with erythropoietic-dependent enzymes than to be the result of hemolysis.

143. The answer is D. *(Robbins, ed 4. pp 146-149.)* The cell in the photomicrograph is known as Gaucher's cell, the pathognomonic histopathologic finding in Gaucher's disease, and is a histiocyte typically found in the spleen, liver, and bone marrow. The cytoplasm contains glucocerebroside in an increased concentration that is demonstrable by periodic acid–Schiff reagent staining and appears wrinkled or striated in ordinary light microscopy. Histochemical ultrastructure studies have revealed that the unique cytoplasmic wrinkles are due to the presence of many spindle-shaped bodies (Gaucher's bodies) that contain 90 percent glucocerebroside and that show increased acid phosphatase activity. A characteristic histopathologic (but not pathognomonic) finding in Niemann-Pick disease is the foam cell; this cell is found mainly in lymphoid tissues.

144. The answer is B. *(Robbins, ed 4. pp 146-149.)* Gaucher's disease is transmitted through an autosomal *recessive* mechanism. The former view that the disease was transmitted through an autosomal *dominant* mechanism was based on erroneous interpretation of the incidence of the disease in several successive generations. The most commonly occurring of the three types of Gaucher's disease is type I. Patients who have this form can expect to live long lives even though symptoms progressively intensify with advancing age.

145. The answer is C. *(Anderson, ed 9. pp 826-827. Robbins, ed 4. pp 695, 1070.)* A woman who manifests a hemorrhagic diathesis following childbirth should be considered to have intravascular coagulopathy until proof to the contrary is obtained—for instance, the condition may be due to retained products of conception. However, the peripheral blood smear depicted in the question shows, in addition to thrombocytopenia (three to four platelets are normally present in every high-power field), remarkably misshaped red blood cells (poikilocytosis) in the form of schistocytes (fragments of red cells), spherocytes, and, importantly, "helmet" red cells, so named because of their similarity in shape to military or football helmets. Helmet cells imply the presence of microangiopathic hemolytic anemia and are thought to form through hemolytic-mechanical red cell membrane disruption by passing through arteriole-capillary beds that have fibrin thrombin meshes. Disorders that cause microangiopathic hemolytic anemia are childhood and adult hemolytic uremic syndrome and thrombotic thrombocytopenic purpura (TTP). The lack of jaundice and neurologic symptoms in this case rules out TTP. The combination of microangiopathic hemolytic anemia and renal insufficiency strongly suggests hemolytic uremic syndrome.

146. The answer is A. *(Robbins, ed 4. pp 666-670.)* Homozygous expression of hemoglobin S results in nearly all the hemoglobin in the red blood cell's being of the S type. Thus, most of the circulating red cells have the abnormal sickling forms that are sequestered by the spleen and produce sludging within the splenic capillaries and consequent multiple and continuing infarctions. Eventually the spleen becomes small as it is replaced by fibrous tissue. This is sometimes referred to as autosplenectomy. Multiple crises contribute to this event. Massive enlargements of the spleen may be found in neoplastic blood disorders. Chronic lymphocytic leukemia (CLL) produces some very large spleens late in the disease, but massive splenomegaly has been seen in many examples of leukemias and lymphomas, including hairy cell leukemia. Even conversion from cutaneous T-cell lymphoma (mycosis fungoides) may result in a transformed immunoblastic-like sarcoma state. The syndrome of myelodyspoiesis also results in splenomegaly.

147. The answer is C. *(Robbins, ed 4. pp 708-711.)* The Rappaport classification has separated NHL into nodular and diffuse categories; this is of major importance since the nodular pattern, independent of the cytologic subtype, is associated with a much better prognosis than is the diffuse type. The nodular lymphomas are composed of neoplastic B cells. Unlike the diffuse lymphomas, which often occur in children and adolescents, nodular lymphomas are rare in those under 20. They affect males and females equally, while diffuse lymphomas are much more common in males. Well-differentiated lymphocytic lymphoma and lymphoblastic lymphoma occur only in the diffuse form.

148. The answer is B. *(Williams, ed 4. p 1069. Wintrobe, ed 8. pp 1708-1709.)* First described by Frizzera in 1974 and subsequently described by Lukes and Tindle, immunoblastic lymphadenopathy (IBL), also called *angioimmunoblastic lymphadenopathy with dysproteinemia,* is an interesting systemic illness. It is characterized by hepatosplenomegaly, skin rash, hemolytic anemia, polyclonal hypergammaglobulinemia, "B" symptoms (including fever and weight loss, with some spontaneous remissions, but often terminating in death), and evolution into immunoblastic sarcoma (rare). The lymph nodes show total effacement of their normal architecture by a diffuse proliferation of plasma cells, lymphoid cells, plasmacytoid cells, and immunoblasts. There is a characteristic proliferation of postcapillary venules, with a type of branching called *arborization* (see photomicrograph). PAS-positive lakes of proteinaceous fluid may also be present in the lymph node. The ultimate prognosis is grim.

149. The answer is E. *(Henry, ed 17. pp 656, 667-668.)* Seen in the photomicrograph are sideroblasts that are demonstrating distinctive rings of Prussian blue–

positive granules that indicate iron. Approximately 35 percent of normoblasts in normal bone marrow contain ferritin granules under normal conditions of iron metabolism. Heme synthetase mediates the attachments of iron onto protoporphyrin for the synthesis of hemoglobin. In sideroblastic anemia the production of globin or of heme is markedly reduced because of the deficiency of pyridoxine and ferritin, which contains iron accumulations with sideroblasts without progression into hemoglobin. The accumulation of these ferritin granules takes place in the mitochondria, where heme synthetase is located, and then can be seen rimming the nucleus of the normoblast—hence the name *ring sideroblasts*. This is the opposite abnormality from iron deficiency anemia. This type of anemia is also referred to as refractory anemia and may be seen in patients suffering from alcoholism, selective deficiencies of pyridoxine, and in malignant conditions such as breast carcinoma.

150. The answer is B. *(Braunwald, ed 11. p 1402.)* The finding of mu heavy-chain proteins in the serum is diagnostic generally of macroglobulinemia and specifically of mu heavy-chain disease. The benign form of macroglobulinemia has been detected in asymptomatic persons without findings of lymphadenopathy, hepatosplenomegaly, anemia, or bone marrow infiltrates of lymphocytes and plasma cells. Increasing levels of the abnormal serum component, onset of bleeding, anemia, or serum hyperviscosity may indicate the need for treatment.

151. The answer is D. *(Robbins, ed 4. pp 737-739.)* Myeloid metaplasia with myelofibrosis is a myeloproliferative disorder in which the bone marrow is hypocellular and fibrotic and extramedullary hematopoiesis occurs, mainly in the spleen (myeloid metaplasia). Marked splenomegaly with trilinear proliferation of normoblasts, immature myeloid cells, and large megakaryocytes occurs. Giant platelets and poikilocytic (teardrop) red cells are seen in the peripheral smear. Clinically, myeloid metaplasia may be preceded by polycythemia vera or chronic myeloid leukemia. Biopsy of the marrow is essential for diagnosis. In contradistinction to chronic myeloid leukemia, levels of leukocyte alkaline phosphatase are elevated or normal in myeloid metaplasia; in CML, levels are low or absent. In 5 to 10 percent of cases of myeloid metaplasia, acute leukemia occurs. In aplastic anemia the marrow is very hypocellular, but consists largely of fat cells, not fibrosis. There is no splenomegaly. Microangiopathic and other hemolytic anemias that result from trauma to red cells show many erythrocytic abnormalities (helmet and burr cells, triangle cells, and schistocytes) in the peripheral smear.

152. The answer is B. *(Robbins, ed 4. p 717.)* T-cell lymphomas occurring in the thoracic cavity in young patients usually arise in the mediastinum and have a particularly aggressive clinical course with rapid growth in the mediastinum impinging upon the trachea or mainstem bronchi and leading to marked respiratory deficiency, which can in turn lead to death in a relatively short period of time if not treated. These unique lymphomas are characterized by rapid cell growth and spread into the circulation, where they produce elevated total white counts reflected by circulating lymphoma cells. As T cells they have characteristics of rosette formation with sheep blood cells. T cells also have subtypes and subsets, which can be delineated by monoclonal antibodies as CD4 helper, CD8 suppressor (cellular differentiation) T-cell surface antigens. The tumor cells also express IL-2 receptor. FC receptors occur on B cells and macrophages. Class II HLA antigens can be found on macrophages, Langerhans cells, and dendritic reticulum cells.

153. The answer is D. *(Robbins, ed 4. pp 686-688.)* Intravascular iron is bound to transferrin, which is usually about 33 percent saturated with iron. Increased saturation occurs in states of iron overload (hemochromatosis), in severe liver disease, hemolytic conditions, and marrow hypoplasia (reduced iron utilization). Iron deficiency is associated with low serum iron levels, increased iron-binding capacity, and decreased saturation.

154. The answer is C. *(Robbins, ed 4. pp 714-715, 718.)* The large-cell immunoblastic lymphoma is one of the three high-grade lymphomas, which also include lymphoblastic lymphoma and small, noncleaved lymphomas, such as Burkitt's lymphoma. Lymphoblastic lymphoma occurs predominantly in adolescents, is closely related to T-cell acute lymphoblastic leukemia, and, in addition to a mediastinal mass, disseminates early to bone marrow and blood. In contrast, large-cell immunoblastic lymphoma is predominantly of B-cell origin (5 to 10 percent are T cell) and occurs in much older people, many of whom had a prior immune or lymphoproliferative disorder (Sjögren's syndrome, AIDS, or renal transplant immunosuppression). Bone marrow involvement is uncommon except in late stages; extranodal tumor (retroperitoneum) is common. The tumor is aggressive and rapidly fatal if untreated. The cells appear plasmacytoid (B immunoblasts) or show multilobed, polymorphous nuclei (T immunoblasts), but molecular studies are essential to differentiate T-cell receptor gene rearrangement from the immunoglobulin gene rearrangements of B immunoblasts.

155. The answer is D. *(Henry, ed 17. pp 684-685.)* Both thalassemia minor and iron deficiency anemia are microcytic disorders in which the mean corpuscular hemoglobin is usually found to be reduced. Red blood cell indexes may be useful in differentiating the two disorders, for while the mean corpuscular hemoglobin concentration (MCHC) is often normal or only slightly reduced in association with thalassemia minor, the MCHC is often definitely reduced in association with iron deficiency anemia. Both pernicious and folate deficiency anemias lead to megaloblastic changes in erythrocytes.

156. The answer is C. *(Robbins, ed 4. pp 261, 288-289, 728-729.)* Chronic myeloid leukemia (CML) is one of the four chronic myeloproliferative disorders, but, unlike myeloid metaplasia or polycythemia vera, CML is associated with the Philadelphia chromosome translocation t (9; 22) in over 90 percent of cases. Association with the translocation t (8; 14) is characteristic of Burkitt's lymphoma. In differentiating CML from a leukemoid reaction, several other features are important: lack of alkaline phosphatase in granulocytes, increased basophils in the peripheral blood, and, often, increased platelets in early stages followed by thrombocytopenia in late or blast stages. Other well-known features of CML include marked splenomegaly, leukocyte counts greater than 50,000/mm^3, and mild anemia.

157. The answer is C. *(Anderson, ed 9. pp 494-495.)* While the exact interactions between different cells is not totally understood, there is current evidence that an initiating antigen is first processed by a macrophage. The macrophage interacts with helper T cells and B cells in a conceptual triangular fashion with helper T cells functioning in the recognition of the carrier component of the antigen on the macrophage as well as recognizing the major histocompatibility complex (MHC) marker (Ia) on the macrophage surface. The macrophage appears to concentrate the antigen, thereby orchestrating interactions between itself and the T and B lymphocytes. After stimulation, the B cell may differentiate into antibody-producing plasma cells. Eosinophils and basophils function in type I reactions (anaphylaxis) by degranulation and binding of IgE.

158. The answer is B. *(Robbins, ed 4. pp 223, 267.)* The findings given are consistent with Wiskott-Aldrich syndrome. The Pelger-Huët anomaly involves leukocytes that have dumbbell-shaped nuclei but function normally. Some of the listed clinical features occur in the Chédiak-Higashi syndrome, but delayed hypersensitivity reactions are normal. In chronic granulomatous disease, leukocytes are unable to kill phagocytized bacteria, but delayed hypersensitivity reactions and platelet counts are normal. In patients who have Hodgkin's disease, a different constellation of symptoms occurs.

159. The answer is D. *(Robbins, ed 4. pp 677-678.)* The autoimmune hemolytic anemias are important causes of acute anemia in a wide variety of clinical states and can be separated into two main types: those secondary to "warm" antibodies and those reactive at cold temperatures. Warm-antibody autoimmune hemolytic anemias react at 37°C in vitro, are composed of IgG, and do not fix complement. They are found in patients with malignant tumors, especially leukemia-lymphoma; with use of such drugs as alpha methyldopa; and in the autoimmune diseases, especially lupus erythematosus. Cold-antibody autoimmune hemolytic anemia reacts at 4 to 6°C, fixes complement, is of the IgM type, and is classically associated with mycoplasma pneumonitis (pleuropneumonia-like organisms). These antibodies are termed *cold agglutinins* and may reach extremely high titers and cause intravascular red cell agglutination.

160. The answer is B (1, 3). *(Robbins, ed 4. pp 717-722.)* The diagnosis of Hodgkin's disease depends on the total histologic picture and the presence of binuclcatcd or bilobcd giant cclls with prominent acidophilic "owl-cyc" nuclcoli known as Reed-Sternberg cells. However, cells similar in appearance to Reed-Sternberg cells may also be seen in infectious mononucleosis, mycosis fungoides, and other conditions. Thus, while Reed-Sternberg cells are necessary to histologically confirm the diagnosis of Hodgkin's lymphoma, they must be present in the appropriate histologic setting of lymphocyte predominance, nodular sclerosis, mixed cellularity, or lymphocyte depletion.

161. The answer is B (1, 3). *(Robbins, ed 4. pp 679-680.)* Macrocytes and hypersegmented neutrophils result from a defect in nuclear maturation within the marrow and are common features of megaloblastic anemia. Myeloblasts would not be seen, and anemia, not polycythemia, would be present.

162. The answer is A (1, 2, 3). *(Robbins, ed 4. pp 681-685.)* The megaloblastic cells shown are larger than normal erythroid precursors and do not show nuclear maturation. They are found in erythroleukemia with myeloblasts, in pernicious anemia, in dietary folate and B_{12} deficiencies, and in patients treated with antimetabolite therapy. Megaloblastic anemias responsive to vitamins B_1, B_6, and C, but not to A, have been reported.

163. The answer is E (all). *(Robbins, ed 4. pp 680-683.)* Although frequently more pronounced in the erythroid series, megaloblastic changes and nuclear abnormalities occur in the myeloid series, including megakaryocytes. A drop in the myeloid-to-erythroid ratio and an increased mitotic rate represent a response to the anemia.

164. The answer is C (2, 4). *(Robbins, ed 4. p 220.)* Serum electrophoresis usually shows only decreased normal immunoglobulins and albumin. Urine electrophoresis followed by immunoelectrophoresis, in contrast, usually reveals a monoclonal spike. Rectal and joint biopsies stained with Congo red and viewed in polarized light are helpful in diagnosis. Dye absorption rates and total dye consumption from the circulation are unreliable.

165. The answer is E (all). *(Williams, ed 4. pp 1151-1153.)* Primary amyloidosis, which is associated with plasma cell dyscrasia, can lead to deposits in all the tissues mentioned and produce the symptoms described. Plasma cell disorders related to primary amyloidosis include classic multiple myeloma, Waldenström's macroglobulinemia, benign monoclonal gammopathy, and nonplasma cell dyscrasias, such as immunodeficiency syndromes and non-Hodgkin's lymphomas. The amyloid found in primary amyloidosis contains immunoglobulin light chain components, whereas the amyloid associated with secondary amyloidosis (chronic disease, such as syphilis, tuberculosis, Whipple's disease, rheumatoid arthritis, Hodgkin's disease, and ulcerative colitis) has no structural similarities to immunoglobulin (AA protein).

166. The answer is C (2, 4). *(Robbins, ed 4. pp 214-215.)* The substance shown is amyloid, with characteristic staining and polarized light appearance. In so-called primary amyloidosis, amyloid is found in patients with multiple myeloma and is usually deposited in all the tissues mentioned. Amyloid deposition to this degree is uncommon in the tongues of elderly people. Primary amyloidosis that accompanies multiple myeloma is most often associated with decreased immunoglobulin levels.

167. The answer is B (1, 3). *(Robbins, ed 4. pp 677-678.)* Erythrocytes that are coated with antierythrocyte antibodies are phagocytized more readily by the reticuloendothelial system than are "normal" erythrocytes. They may also be lysed directly by complement. Autoimmune antibodies may be either warm-acting (IgG) or reactive at 5°C (cold agglutinins).

168. The answer is B (1, 3). *(Robbins, ed 4. pp 717-722.)* Successful treatment of Hodgkin's disease (HD) continues to be the rule, although a few patients have not had the usual dramatic response to therapy. HD is classified as having lymphocyte predominance, lymphocyte depletion, nodular sclerosis, or mixed cellularity according to the histologic appearance. Reed-Sternberg cells, which are the characteristic, large, binucleated cells with prominent nucleoli, are more numerous in the mixed cellularity and nodular sclerosis types and are rare in lymphocyte predominance. Since newer protocols for the treatment of HD even in advanced stages (stages III and IV) are yielding dramatic responses, some workers report their results on overall HD cases without regard to the histologic subtype. The overall prognosis for all HD cases in the United States in 1985 can be said to be relatively very good, and the less common lymphocyte predominance subtype carries an excellent prognosis. The letter "A" attached to the stage number means the patient is asymptomatic and is not anemic, whereas "B" denotes the presence of pruritus, fever, weight loss, and anemia. "Stage I" means that there is lymph node involvement in one region only; "stage II" means that the lymph nodes involved are on the same side of the diaphragm; "stage III" means that both sides of the diaphragm are involved (if the spleen is involved, the letter "s" is affixed); and "stage IV" involves dissemination to extralymphatic tissue, such as bone marrow, liver, and lung.

169. The answer is E (all). *(Williams, ed 4. pp 189-190.)* Paroxysmal nocturnal hemoglobinuria (PNH) is a rare example of chronic hemolytic anemia in which intravascular hemolysis occurs because of an intrinsic membrane abnormality of erythrocytes, an idiopathic acquired defect of young adults who have complement-sensitive red cells. There is often a pancytopenia. Hemosiderinuria occurs in all cases, although nocturnal hemoglobinuria is found in a minority. Venous thromboses are a frequent complication (Budd-Chiari syndrome from hepatic vein thrombosis). PNH may arise de novo, or follow an episode of aplastic anemia, so the possible existence of PNH must be considered in a patient presenting with aplastic anemia. Laboratory findings in PNH include hemosiderinuria, hemolysis by dilute sucrose solution (sucrose hemolysis test), and a positive acid-serum lysis (Ham acid hemolysis) test.

170-174. The answers are: 170-C, 171-C, 172-D, 173-A, 174-B. *(Robbins, ed 4. pp 724-730.)* Auer rods are often prominent in the hypergranular promyelocytes of acute promyelocytic leukemia since they are formed from the abnormal azurophilic granules. Myeloblasts predominate in acute myeloblastic leukemia (AML) and, therefore, only a few granules, or occasional Auer rods, are present. Acute pro-myelocytic leukemia is associated with a short course and widespread petechiae and ecchymoses, cutaneous or mucosal, from disseminated intravascular coagulation. The M1 and M3 classes refer to the French-American-British (FAB) classification of AML: M1 is AML in which myeloblasts predominate and M3 is acute promye-locytic leukemia with promyelocytes numerous. Myeloperoxidase is present in both, especially in M3. AML occasionally follows chemotherapy and radiotherapy for Hodgkin's disease.

Chronic lymphocytic leukemia occurs most frequently after the age of 50 (90 percent of cases). It is associated with long survival in many cases and the few symptoms are related to anemia and the absolute lymphocytosis of small mature cells. Splenomegaly may be noted. Some patients are asymptomatic.

Acute lymphoblastic leukemia (ALL) affects children and young adults with marked lymphadenopathy, some splenomegaly, and hepatomegaly. Since chemo-therapy at present results in complete remission in 90 percent of children, with more than 50 percent alive 5 years later, it is essential to differentiate ALL from acute myeloblastic leukemia in which prognosis is poor. Cytochemical differentiation includes PAS-positive blasts in most cases of ALL and the presence of terminal deoxynucleotidyl transferase (TdT) in 95 percent of cases of ALL, but in less than 5 percent of acute myeloblastic leukemias.

Hairy cell leukemia and chronic lymphocytic leukemia (CLL) are considered to be chronic lymphoproliferative disorders. CLL is a neoplasm of B cells, like most other lymphoid malignancies. Through molecular analysis, hairy cells are now known to rearrange and express immunoglobulin genes, assigning them also to B-cell lineage.

Cardiovascular System

DIRECTIONS: Each question below contains five suggested responses. Select the **one best** response to each question.

175. An 82-year-old woman complaining of headaches, visual disturbances, and muscle pain has a biopsy of the temporal artery. The changes revealed by the biopsy specimen are shown in the photomicrograph below. The next course of action is to

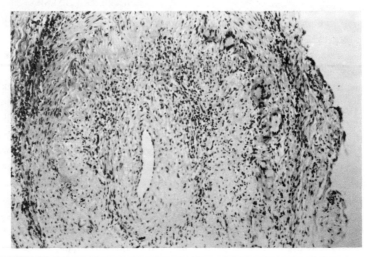

(A) administer corticosteroids
(B) verify with a repeat biopsy
(C) administer anticoagulants
(D) perform angiography
(E) order an ESR test

176.. If the coronary arteries on dissection at autopsy show severe atherosclerosis in a patient who had clinical acute (60-hour) myocardial infarction, you would expect to find

(A) definite gross evidence of infarction
(B) coronary thrombosis in 90 percent of cases
(C) coronary thrombosis in 65 percent of cases
(D) a plaque with ulceration, fissure, or hemorrhage
(E) rupture of a papillary muscle

177. Complete obliteration of the aortic lumen by a coarctation proximal to the ductus arteriosus is fatal unless

(A) the foramen ovale is closed
(B) the ductus is ligated
(C) pulmonary stenosis coexists
(D) the ductus remains patent
(E) the tricuspid valve is incompetent

178. Which of the following conditions is most likely to predispose to thrombosis and embolism?

(A) Atrial fibrillation
(B) Pulmonary stenosis
(C) Ventricular septal defect
(D) Aortic stenosis
(E) Atrial septal defect

179. Features of Fallot's tetralogy include all the following EXCEPT

(A) obstruction to the pulmonary outflow
(B) hypertrophy of the right ventricle
(C) aortic dextroposition in 50 percent of cases
(D) cyanosis developing before 1 year of age
(E) ventricular septal defect

180. The form of vascular disease responsible for malignant hypertension is

(A) medial calcific sclerosis
(B) arteriosclerosis obliterans
(C) hyperplastic arteriolosclerosis
(D) hyaline arteriolosclerosis
(E) thromboangiitis obliterans

181. The most common cause of infectious myocarditis is

(A) diphtheritic infection
(B) Coxsackie viral infection
(C) Chagas' disease
(D) trichinosis
(E) brucellosis

182. The mortality from myocardial infarction is most closely related to the occurrence of

(A) a pericardial effusion
(B) pulmonary edema
(C) coronary artery thrombosis
(D) an arrhythmia
(E) systemic hypotension

183. A synonym for *nonbacterial thrombotic endocarditis* is

(A) atypical verrucous endocarditis
(B) marantic endocarditis
(C) Libman-Sacks endocarditis
(D) viridans endocarditis
(E) none of the above

184. An elderly man treated for congestive heart failure for years with digitalis and furosemide dies of pulmonary edema. A postmortem examination of the heart would most likely show

(A) severe left ventricular hypertrophy
(B) right and left ventricular hypertrophy
(C) right ventricular infarction
(D) aortic and mitral valve stenosis
(E) a dilated, globular heart with thin walls

185. The pathology evident in the photomicrograph below usually first appears after which of the following lengths of time following a myocardial infarction?

(A) 12 hours
(B) 3 days
(C) 7 days
(D) 14 days
(E) 28 days

186. The photomicrograph below depicts the presence of

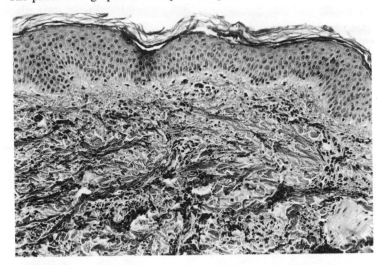

(A) disseminated candidiasis
(B) pigmented purpuric dermatosis
(C) anaphylactoid purpura (leukocytoclastic angiitis)
(D) erythema multiforme
(E) reaction to the bite of an arthropod

187. Manifestations of rheumatic fever that are of major diagnostic value include all the following EXCEPT

(A) subcutaneous nodules
(B) migratory arthritis of large joints
(C) fever
(D) erythema marginatum
(E) chorea minor

188. A 9-year-old boy is seen in the emergency room with severe, colicky abdominal pain, a purpuric rash, evidence of polyarthralgia, and hematuria. The mother considers these signs and symptoms to be the aftermath of an upper respiratory infection the boy had some time previously. A skin biopsy of the rash would most likely show

(A) no abnormalities
(B) viral vesicles
(C) leukocytoclastic vasculitis (angiitis)
(D) hyaline thrombi
(E) scabies mites

189. Lipofuscin most characteristically accumulates

(A) in glycogen storage disease
(B) in the renal tubular epithelium
(C) in a perinuclear distribution
(D) as a consequence of hemolysis
(E) from extrahepatic obstruction

190. Bacterial endocarditis constitutes the greatest threat to patients who have which of the following forms of congenital heart disease?

(A) Atrial septal defect
(B) Ventricular septal defect
(C) Pulmonic stenosis
(D) Tetralogy of Fallot
(E) Patent ductus arteriosus

191. A 56-year-old woman died in a hospital where she was being evaluated for shortness of breath, ankle edema, and mild hepatomegaly. Because of the gross appearance of the liver at necropsy in the photograph below, one would also expect to find

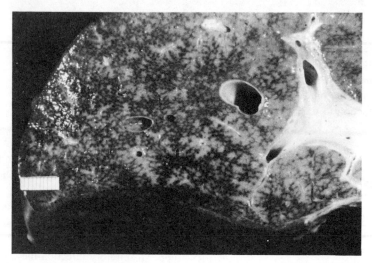

(A) a pulmonary saddle embolus
(B) right heart dilatation
(C) portal vein thrombosis
(D) biliary cirrhosis
(E) splenic amyloidosis

192. The necrotizing inflammation of the small gastrointestinal artery shown in the photomicrograph below is most likely due to

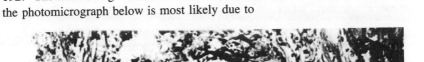

(A) myasthenia gravis
(B) polyarteritis nodosa
(C) atherosclerosis
(D) dissecting aneurysm
(E) syphilis

DIRECTIONS: Each question below contains four suggested responses of which **one or more** is correct. Select

A	if	**1, 2, and 3**	are correct
B	if	**1 and 3**	are correct
C	if	**2 and 4**	are correct
D	if	**4**	is correct
E	if	**1, 2, 3, and 4**	are correct

193. The biopsy specimen shown below reveals a dermal vascular tumor with angular, slitlike spaces and spindle cells in the dermal stroma. This lesion is associated with

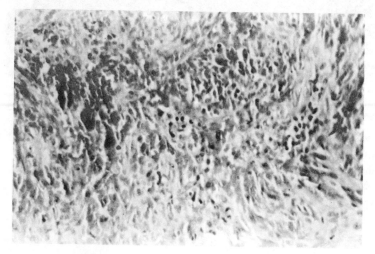

(1) four clinically distinct forms
(2) intestinal bleeding
(3) early histologic resemblance to dermatitis
(4) tumor origin from vascular endothelium

194. Myocardial rupture as a consequence of myocardial infarction

(1) results from long-standing ventricular aneurysm
(2) rarely occurs after the third week
(3) correlates with previous left ventricular hypertrophy
(4) most likely results in tamponade

195. Severe mitral stenosis, as shown in the photograph below, is frequently accompanied by

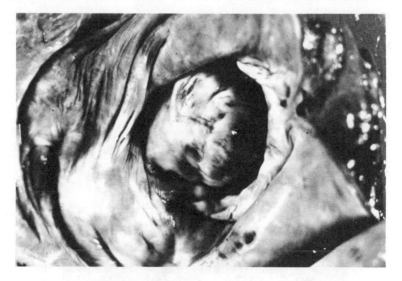

(1) severe left ventricular hypertrophy
(2) left atrial enlargement with atrial fibrillation
(3) pulmonary valvular stenosis
(4) chronic passive pulmonary congestion

196. Isolated granulomatous myocarditis is also known as

(1) idiopathic myocarditis
(2) sarcoid myocarditis
(3) Fiedler's myocarditis
(4) Friedreich's ataxia myocarditis

197. Acute infective endocarditis differs from subacute endocarditis in which of the following respects?

(1) The time required for the lesion to develop
(2) The nature of the preponderant organism
(3) Embolization and dissemination
(4) The nature of valvular vegetations

198. A 36-year-old man with a long history of cigarette smoking is being evaluated for nausea, sweating, and substernal pressure discomfort. Which of the following determinations would be helpful in excluding an acute myocardial infarction?

(1) Isoenzymes of creatine phosphokinase (CPK)
(2) Serum glutamic oxaloacetic transaminase (SGOT, AST)
(3) Lactic dehydrogenase isoenzymes (LDH)
(4) Isoenzymes of alkaline phosphatase

SUMMARY OF DIRECTIONS

A	B	C	D	E
1, 2, 3 only	1, 3 only	2, 4 only	4 only	All are correct

199. Tumors known for involvement of the atrium include

(1) metastatic fibrosarcoma
(2) primary myxoma
(3) metastatic colon carcinoma
(4) renal cell carcinoma

200. The heart in the gross photograph below came from a patient who

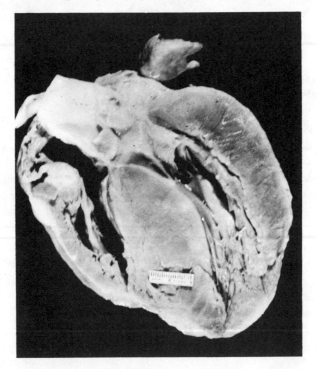

(1) may have experienced sudden, unexpected death
(2) had Libman-Sacks endocarditis
(3) may have had a family history of similar cardiac involvement
(4) frequently had obstructive symptoms

201. Cardiac involvement has been linked to which of the following conditions?

(1) Hemochromatosis
(2) Rocky Mountain spotted fever
(3) Sarcoidosis
(4) Breast carcinoma

202. Cardiac lesions occurring in ankylosing spondylitis closely resemble those of

(1) rheumatic myocarditis
(2) rheumatoid heart disease
(3) syphilitic myocarditis
(4) syphilitic aortitis

DIRECTIONS: Each group of questions below consists of lettered headings followed by a set of numbered items. For each numbered item select the **one** lettered heading with which it is **most** closely associated. Each lettered heading may be used **once, more than once, or not at all.**

Questions 203-206

Match the following descriptive phrases with the appropriate lettered type of cardiomyopathy.

(A) Hypertrophic cardiomyopathy
(B) Dilated (congestive) cardio-myopathy
(C) Constrictive (restrictive) cardiomyopathy
(D) Secondary cardiomyopathy
(E) Endomyocardial fibrosis

203. Thirty percent of patients are prone to sudden cardiac death

204. May develop in patients with multiple myeloma

205. Obstruction of left ventricular outflow of blood

206. Usually identified in Southeast Asia and Africa

Questions 207-210

For each cardiac condition choose the infectious agent with which it is most likely to be associated.

(A) Coxsackievirus
(B) *Mycobacterium tuberculosis*
(C) *Streptococcus*
(D) *Treponema*
(E) *Escherichia coli*

207. Primary myocarditis

208. Rheumatic fever

209. Aortic aneurysms

210. Suppurative pericarditis

Questions 211-214

For each aneurysm, choose the disease or syndrome with which it is most likely to be associated.

(A) Ehlers-Danlos syndrome
(B) Kawasaki's disease
(C) Rheumatic disease
(D) Polycystic renal disease
(E) Takayasu's arteritis

211. Berry aneurysm

212. Dissecting aortic aneurysm

213. Coronary aneurysm

214. Abdominal and distal thoracic aortic aneurysms

Questions 215-217

Match each of the gross or microscopic cardiac alterations below with the most appropriate disease.

(A) Myxedema
(B) Addison's disease
(C) Beriberi
(D) Carcinoid syndrome
(E) Fatty degeneration

215. Fibrosis of tricuspid and pulmonary valves

216. Globose heart

217. "Thrush-breast" myocardium

Cardiovascular System
Answers

175. The answer is A. *(Robbins, ed 4. pp 574-576.)* Giant cell arteritis (temporal arteritis), although not a major public-health problem, is an important disease to consider in the differential diagnosis of patients of middle to advanced age who present with a constellation of symptoms that may include migratory muscular and back pains (polymyalgia rheumatica), dizziness, visual disturbances, headaches, weight loss, anorexia, and tenderness over one or both of the temporal arteries. The cause of the arteritis (which may include giant cells, neutrophils, and chronic inflammatory cells) is unknown, but the dramatic response to corticosteroids suggests an immunogenic origin. The disease may involve any artery within the body, but involvement of the ophthalmic artery or arteries may lead to blindness unless steroid therapy is begun. Therefore, if clinically suspected, the workup to document temporal arteritis should be expedited and should include a biopsy of the temporal artery. Frequently, the erythrocyte sedimentation rate (ESR) is markedly elevated to values of 90 or greater. Whereas tenderness, nodularity, or skin reddening over the course of one of the scalp arteries, particularly the temporal, may show the ideal portion for a biopsy, it is important to recognize that temporal arterial segments may be segmentally uninvolved or not involved at all even when the disease is present.

176. The answer is D. *(Robbins, ed 4. pp 564, 606-608.)* At autopsy, coronary artery thrombosis has been found in less than 50 percent of cases of myocardial infarction (MI). However, when coronary angiography is done within 4 hours of MI onset, a thrombosed artery is found in almost 90 percent of cases; occlusion is found in only about 60 percent when angiography is delayed for 12 to 24 hours. Therefore, lysis occurs or there is relaxation of spasm, or both. Also, intravenous or intracoronary fibrinolysins restore flow to thrombosed arteries in more than 75 percent of recent MIs. These findings are proof of coronary thrombosis, whether it is found at autopsy or not. Ulcerated, fissured, or hemorrhagic atheromas are usually found beneath the thrombus, whether still attached or lysed.

177. The answer is D. *(Robbins, ed 4. pp 624-625.)* Coarctation of the aorta occurs in 6 to 14 percent of cases of congenital heart disease. In its infantile form, coarctation takes place in the root of the aorta proximal to the ductus arteriosus, which, if patent, serves as a bypass to allow blood flow to the arterial system. Usually, surgical intervention is necessary for infants who have this anomaly, which may cause death soon after birth or within the first year of life.

178. The answer is A. *(Robbins, ed 4. pp 99-106.)* Stasis of blood in fibrillating atria predisposes to thrombosis and embolism. Systemic embolization from left atrial thrombi may cause infarction in the brain, lower extremities, spleen, and kidneys. Endocardial mural thrombi occur as a consequence of myocardial infarction, bacterial endocarditis, or nonbacterial (marantic) endocarditis.

179. The answer is C. *(Braunwald, ed 11. pp 949-950.)* Fallot's tetralogy consists of subaortic ventricular septal defect, obstruction to right ventricular outflow, aortic override of the ventricular septal defect, and moderate right ventricular hypertrophy. The obstruction to right ventricular outflow may be caused by infundibular stenosis of the right ventricle or stenosis of the pulmonic valve. A right-sided aorta occurs in about 25 percent of cases with tetralogy. Most patients are cyanotic from birth or develop cyanosis by the end of the first year of life, since even mild obstruction to right ventricular outflow is progressive. Tetralogy of Fallot is the most common cause of cyanosis after 1 year of age and causes 10 percent of all forms of congenital heart disease. Hypoxic attacks and syncope are serious complications, forming the commonest mode of death from this disease during infancy and childhood. Other complications include infectious endocarditis, paradoxical embolism, polycythemia, and cerebral infarction or abscess.

180. The answer is C. *(Robbins, ed 4. pp 569-570, 577.) Malignant hypertension* refers to dramatic elevations in systolic and diastolic blood pressure often resulting in early death from cerebral and brainstem hemorrhages. Pathologically the renal vessels demonstrate a concentric obliteration of arterioles by an increase in smooth muscle cells, and protein deposition in a laminar configuration that includes fibrin material, which leads to total and subtotal occlusion of the vessels. Hyaline arteriolosclerosis as seen in diabetes is presumably caused by leakage of plasma components across the endothelium with or without hypertension. Medial calcific sclerosis (Mönckeberg's arteriosclerosis) is characterized by dystrophic calcification in the tunica media of muscular arteries. Thromboangiitis obliterans (Buerger's disease) is occlusion by a proliferative inflammatory process in arteries of heavy cigarette smokers and is often associated with HLA-A9, B5 genotypes.

181. The answer is B. *(Anderson, ed 9. pp 659-664. Robbins, ed 4. pp 640-643.)* Although numerous agents—bacterial, protozoal, fungal, or parasitic—are causative of infectious myocarditis, the most common type is viral myocarditis, which often presents as a primary infection. The Coxsackie viral group, principally Coxsackie B, is most often implicated. Coxsackie myocarditis in children is often preceded by upper respiratory tract infection. Other viral diseases in which myocarditis occurs include rubella and polio. Chagas' disease (*Trypanosoma cruzi*) is also prominent as a cause of myocarditis in endemic areas of South America, where up to half the population is infected. Bacterial myocarditis is not common, but the diphtheria bacillus is causative through its exotoxin (toxic myocarditis). The bacteria of brucellosis, tularemia, and tuberculosis produce small granulomas within the myocardium. *Trichinella spiralis* larvae frequently penetrate myocardial fibers; they do not encyst, but interstitial myocarditis may result.

182. The answer is D. *(Robbins, ed 4. pp 612-614.)* In myocardial infarction, life-threatening arrhythmias occur in approximately 45 percent of patients without shock and in more than 90 percent of patients with shock. The most common arrhythmias are expressed as ventricular extrasystoles, but atrial extrasystoles, sinus tachycardia, and sinus bradycardia also occur. Even without arrhythmias, nearly two-thirds of patients with acute myocardial infarcts develop heart failure and pulmonary edema. Sudden death (death within 24 hours of onset of symptoms and signs) occurs in about 20 to 25 percent of acute attacks.

183. The answer is B. *(Anderson, ed 9. pp 652-655.)* Nonbacterial thrombotic endocarditis is a form of endocarditis involving the mitral and aortic valves especially, characterized by resemblance to the verrucous-like protuberances of rheumatic valvulitis, which are usually large and friable; smooth and polypoid and shaggy forms are also encountered. These also may resemble the vegetations of bacterial endocarditis, but the lesions are sterile and contain no microorganisms. Both surfaces of the valves are not involved, as they may be in Libman-Sacks or atypical verrucous endocarditis. *Viridans endocarditis* is a synonym for *subacute bacterial endocarditis.* Nonbacterial thrombotic endocarditis is also referred to as *terminal* or *marantic endocarditis* and is associated in this country with advanced stages of cachexia as is found in advanced stages of malignancy or starvation. It occurs in many other terminal wasting diseases but has recently been described in well-nourished persons who have died acutely; thus, the older terms *marantic* and *terminal* are probably not appropriate. The pathogenesis is not clear, although there is evidence for increased coagulability in some patients, and the disorder may be associated with disseminated intravascular coagulation.

184. The answer is E. *(Robbins, ed 4. pp 598-601.)* The morphologic changes of clinical congestive heart failure cannot always be correlated with necropsy findings of the heart because there may be hypertrophy, dilatation, a combination of both, or even an absence of both. Many patients with long-standing congestive heart failure after decompensation will have hearts that are maximally dilated, with thinned and unusually soft myocardium rather than hypertrophic ventricular myocardium. This thinning of the myocardium occurs after a long period of compensatory hypertrophy and reflects a state in which the capacity of the myocardium to compensate has been exceeded. The first response of the myocardium to a demand for increased work (load) is to undergo hypertrophy according to Starling's law, leading to an increase in stroke volume. Eventually, this mechanism is exceeded under states of increased oxygen demand or demand for more cardiac output, and cardiac decompensation results, with the worst complication being acute pulmonary edema as a consequence of left ventricular failure.

185. The answer is B. *(Robbins, ed 4. pp 609-611.)* Usually by 3 days after a myocardial infarction, the predominant microscopic features that develop and that can be seen in a stained section of the affected myocardium include coagulation necrosis of fibers and evidence of extensive neutrophilic exudation. Interstitial edema may also be observed in microscopy, and the cross-striations of fibers may appear less recognizable. In gross examination 3 days after the infarction, the infarct has a hyperemic border surrounding a central portion that is yellow-brown and soft as the result of fatty change.

186. The answer is C. *(Robbins, ed 4. pp 573-574.)* Anaphylactoid purpura (also known as leukocytoclastic or hypersensitivity angiitis) is characterized clinically by palpable purpura in patients reacting to an antigen derived from drugs (especially the semisynthetic penicillins), from infections (including beta-streptococcal pharyngitis), and possibly from neoplasms. Pathologically, the epidermis is generally intact with vascular damage in the form of fibrinoid necrosis and occlusion of these small capillaries, venules, and arterioles of the dermis by fibrin and proteinaceous deposits, which may include IgA and complement. Hallmarks of the disease histologically are neutrophils that extend out from the damaged vessels and show karyorrhexis (nuclear dust). Extravasated red cells are also seen. Disseminated candidiasis is characterized by varying degrees of severity of epidermal micropustules, folliculitis, or dermal abscesses. Erythema multiforme generally presents with epidermal cell necrosis, an inflammatory cell infiltrate in the dermis, and bullae separating the epidermis from the dermis. Arthropod reactions may have polymorphic inflammatory cells that include neutrophils, eosinophils, macrophages, and lymphocytes, but lymphocytic hyperplasia is frequently the hallmark in the hypersensitivity chronic form.

187. The answer is C. *(Robbins, ed 4. pp 629-633.)* Rheumatic fever (RF) is a systemic disease with the major findings of migratory polyarthritis of large joints, carditis, erythema marginatum of skin (although skin involvement is not very common), subcutaneous nodules, and Sydenham's chorea, a neurologic disorder with involuntary, purposeless, rapid movements, most likely to occur in adolescent females and during pregnancy. There is no relation to Huntington's chorea. Fever is a minor characterization, although quite frequent. Rheumatic nodules may develop over pressure points during the later stages and seldom occur in cases without cardiac involvement. RF usually follows a pharyngeal infection with group A β-hemolytic streptococci because of an autoimmune mechanism based on cross-reactions between cardiac antigens and antibodies evoked by one of the many streptococcal antigens, e.g., streptococcal M protein. Immunofluorescence shows immunoglobulins and complement along sarcolemmal sheaths of cardiac myofibers, but Aschoff bodies seldom contain immunoglobulins or complement.

188. The answer is C. *(Robbins, ed 4. pp 573-574, 692, 1043-1044.)* The development of apparent multiple-system involvement (e.g., of the gastrointestinal tract and the skeletal, renal, and cutaneous systems) by an obscure agent, preceded by an upper respiratory tract infection, should arouse suspicion of hypersensitivity angiitis (Henoch-Schönlein purpura). This syndrome is characterized by a generalized vasculitis distinct from other types of vasculitis, such as Wegener's granulomatosis and polyarteritis nodosa, in that a simple, superficial skin biopsy of the rash demonstrates an acute inflammatory infiltrate of the upper dermal small vessels and capillaries with degenerating neutrophils (karyorrhexis) and extravasated red cells. This form of superficial vasculitis is termed *leukocytoclastic vasculitis;* its presence in the clinical setting just described enables one to make a diagnosis. Gastrointestinal hemorrhages presumably result from a similar involvement of the vessels in the mucosa. The glomerular mesangium may contain deposits of complement, fibrin, and IgA.

189. The answer is C. *(Anderson, ed 9. pp 34, 35, 43.)* Lipofuscin consists of insoluble lipid pigment. It occurs in the cells of organs and is demonstrated by a brown intracellular pigment deposition that can occur in a wide variety of cell types. It is predominantly seen in the United States in the liver and myocardium of elderly persons and is characteristically deposited in a perinuclear distribution. Lipofuscin also may result from malnutrition or any disease that causes chronic wasting in other age groups. It represents the accumulation of nondigested material within the cell lysosomes. So much lipofuscin may be deposited in an organ itself (e.g., in the heart) that the organ may appear grossly brown. Increased bilirubin results from hemolysis of red blood cells as well as obstructive jaundice. The pigmentation appears yellow to yellow-green.

190. The answer is B. *(Robbins, ed 4. pp 633-637.)* Even though children and infants who have small isolated ventricular septal defects are usually asymptomatic, and even though two-thirds of infants who have uncomplicated lesions will have spontaneous closure of their ventricular septal defects by the age of 5, the main risk for these patients is bacterial endocarditis. Protection against bacteremia with antibiotics during routine but potentially infectious procedures is therefore required.

191. The answer is B. *(Robbins, ed 4. pp 600-601.)* The photograph shows the classic pattern of hepatic congestion around central veins, which leads to necrosis and degeneration of the hepatocytes surrounded by pale peripheral residual parenchyma. This is the pattern arising in the liver from chronic passive congestion as a result of right heart failure (termed "nutmeg liver"). Mitral stenosis with consequent pulmonary hypertension leads to right heart failure, as does any cause of pulmonary hypertension, such as emphysema (cor pulmonale). Right heart failure also leads to congestion of the spleen and transudation of fluid into the abdomen (ascites) and lower extremity soft tissues (pitting ankle edema) as a result of venous congestion. Portal vein thrombosis is most often seen in association with hepatic cirrhosis.

192. The answer is B. *(Robbins, ed 4. pp 571-573.)* Polyarteritis nodosa, as a necrotizing inflammation that occurs in episodes at random locations within or on the walls of medium-sized and small arteries, has been reported in about 0.1 percent of autopsies and affects, in order of increasing frequency, the arteries associated with peripheral and central nerves, skeletal muscles, pancreas, gastrointestinal tract, liver, heart, and kidneys. Proceeding in stages, the inflammatory reaction features acute necrosis, with fibrinoid deposition and neutrophilic infiltration, and leads to thrombosis of the lumen and destruction of the internal elastic membrane. Polyarteritis nodosa probably could be more accurately called "panarteritis nodosa," because *all* vascular coats are subject to inflammation. A remnant of the internal elastic membrane is visible in the photomicrograph.

193. The answer is E (all). *(Robbins, ed 4. pp 591-592, 1291-1292.)* Kaposi's sarcoma (KS) comprises four distinct forms. The classic, or European, form has been known since 1862. It occurs in older men of Eastern European or Mediterranean origin (predominantly Italian or Jewish) and is characterized by purple maculopapular skin lesions of the lower extremities and visceral involvement in only 10 percent of cases. The African form occurs in younger people and is more aggressive; it often involves lymph nodes in children. The rare form in immunosuppressed recipients of renal transplants often regresses when immunosuppression stops. In the epidemic form associated with AIDS, skin lesions may occur anywhere and include dissemination to mucous membranes, GI tract, lymph nodes, and viscera. Histologic determination is difficult, but all four clinical types appear similar. Early, irregular, dilated epidermal vascular spaces, extravasated red cells, and hemosiderin (like granulation tissue or stasis dermatitis) are characteristic. Later, more characteristic lesions show spindle cells around slit-spaces that are angular and contain red cells—a picture like that of angiosarcoma. The tumor cells are almost certainly of vascular endothelial origin (blood vessel or lymphatic or both). This often multifocal disease is rarely fatal, but death may be caused by frequent opportunistic infections or, less often, lymphoma, leukemia, or myeloma.

194. The answer is C (2, 4). *(Anderson, ed 9. pp 638-639.)* Myocardial rupture as a consequence of acute myocardial infarction occurs in 5 to 25 percent of cases of acute infarct, depending on the series reported. Actual rupture of the myocardium is related to the softening of the myocardial wall and occurs usually within the first week of onset of the infarction when there is maximal softening caused by necrosis. It rarely is seen after the third week, at which time fibrosis is taking place. It is seen not uncommonly in females, especially those with preexisting hypertension. More commonly it occurs through the free wall of the left ventricle, in which case cardiac tamponade is produced by massive blood volume displacement into the pericardial sac, which is constrained by its limits of expansibility. This complication occurs in about 70 percent of cases.

195. The answer is C (2, 4). *(Anderson, ed 9. pp 672-673.)* Mitral stenosis is most often associated with aortic valve disease and occasionally with tricuspid valve disease, especially in people with antecedent rheumatic fever. Occasionally, both aortic and mitral disease result from atherosclerosis. Pulmonary valvular stenosis is rarely caused by either aortic or mitral disease. Since severe mitral stenosis prevents significant regurgitation, left ventricular enlargement would not be expected. Left atrial enlargement and chronic pulmonary congestion are common in mitral disease.

196. The answer is B (1, 3). *(Anderson, ed 9. pp 662-664.)* Idiopathic myocarditis is also known as Fiedler's myocarditis and isolated myocarditis because the inflammation is limited to the myocardium and does not involve the endocardial surfaces, valves, or pericardium. This form of myocarditis may take two forms: a diffuse type consisting of nonspecific lymphocytes, macrophages, eosinophils, rare neutrophils, and plasma cells that are distributed throughout the interstitium of the heart; and a type that is characterized by a granulomatous inflammation with multinucleated giant cells of the foreign body and of the Langhans' type. No caseation is seen in the granulomatous form and acid-fast bacilli microorganisms are not present. While sarcoidosis may involve the heart with noncaseating granulomas, at the present time idiopathic myocarditis is not thought to be related to sarcoidosis. Sudden death may occur in Fiedler's myocarditis. Friedreich's ataxia produces myocardial fibrosis and degeneration of myocardial fibers with a few lymphocytes but is not related to Fiedler's myocarditis.

197. The answer is A (1, 2, 3). *(Robbins, ed 4. pp 633-637.)* Infective endocarditis, unlike rheumatic endocarditis, continues to be a clinical problem even in the antibiotic era, with such new factors as intravenous drug abuse and immunosuppression contributing to its persistence. The successful outcome of treatment is directly dependent on early recognition and diagnosis, since with time the infective organisms (such as yeast, bacteria, rickettsiae) tend to be covered with fibrin and platelets, thereby preventing access of antibiotics to the organisms. In addition, delayed treatment allows time for local valvular destruction. Acute endocarditis (AC) tends to develop within days on previously normal valves (60 percent of cases), whereas subacute endocarditis (SEC) takes more time to develop, may be clinically silent, and may be manifested only by the patient complaining of "not being up to par." The organism causing AC tends to be pathogenic (e.g., *Staphylococcus aureus* or gonococcus); the organism causing SEC tends to be relatively innocuous (e.g., microaerophilic streptococci, *Streptococcus viridans*, and even diphtheroids). Bacterial embolization from the valves to other organs occurs mainly in AC and is much less common in SEC. Despite small differences, such as the smaller vegetations occurring in SEC than in AC, it is not usually possible to distinguish SEC vegetations from AC vegetations through only structural criteria.

198. The answer is B (1, 3). *(Henry, ed 17. pp 254, 273. Robbins, ed 4. pp 612-613.)* The isoenzymes of creatine phosphokinase (CPK) and lactic dehydrogenase

(LDH) are the most helpful in assessing myocardial necrosis accurately. Total LDH values are not useful unless the isoenzyme levels have been determined, since LDH is notoriously nonspecific and is widespread in mammalian cells. The highest levels of total LDH, for example, are found in hypoxemic shock, megaloblastic anemia, and widespread carcinomatosis. LDH can be separated into five fractions by electrophoresis; if the LD_1 fraction is greater than the LD_2 fraction ("flipped pattern"), this is characteristic of myocardial necrosis. CPK can also be separated into its isoenzyme fractions, with an elevated MB fraction indicating myocardial necrosis. Both the LD_1 and CPK-MB fractions are elevated within 10 to 22 hours of necrosis. SGOT (aspartate transaminase, or AST) lacks specificity, since it may leak out of the cells that have not undergone necrosis and its levels may be elevated in pulmonary infarction and liver disease. Alkaline phosphatase levels are elevated in liver disease and metabolic bone disease.

199. The answer is C (2, 4). *(Robbins, ed 4. pp 651-653.)* Primary myxomas of the heart may involve all four chambers; however, there is a propensity for involving the left atrium in a ratio of 3:1 to 4:1. They may be small or large, are attached to the endocardial surface, and often produce a ball-valve action. Portions of them can fragment and embolize to skin, brain, and other organs. Renal cell carcinoma has been known to penetrate the renal vein, which drains the kidney harboring the tumor and extends into the inferior vena cava, and thereby gain access to the right atrium. On rare occasions cardiac symptoms caused by the renal vein extension of renal carcinoma may be the first sign of the tumor. Recently it has been shown that cardiac myxomas may be associated with a familial syndrome that combines cardiac myxomas with cutaneous lentigines, pigmented nodular hyperplasia of the adrenal glands, and Leydig cell tumors. Colon carcinoma may manifest widespread dissemination, but the organ of metastatic involvement is usually the liver. When fibrosarcoma disseminates, it does so by the circulatory system with its favorite site being the lungs.

200. The answer is B (1, 3). *(Robbins, ed 4. pp 644-646.)* The cardiomyopathy shown in the photograph is designated *hypertrophic cardiomyopathy* with the synonyms of *idiopathic hypertrophic subaortic stenosis (IHSS), hypertrophic obstructive cardiomyopathy,* and *asymmetric septal hypertrophy (ASH).* It is characterized by a prominent and hypertrophic interventricular septum that is out of proportion to the thickness of the left ventricle. Histologically the myocardial fibers have disarray caused by wide fibers with unusual orientation, and prominent hyperchromatic nuclei. There is increased incidence within families and there is evidence that it may be an autosomal dominant disorder. Patients may have dyspnea, light-headedness, and chest pain, especially upon physical exertion; however, many patients appear to be asymptomatic although a sudden, unexpected death occurs not infrequently, especially following or during physical exertion. There may be abnormalities of the coronary arteries. The mitral valve may be thickened and patients may experience endocarditis on it. Cardiac output can be markedly reduced in some patients because of reduced volume of the left ventricle. As the patient ages, however, cardiac dilatation often improves the reduced left ventricular volume.

201. The answer is E (all). *(Anderson, ed 9. pp 660-661, 686, 704-705.)* The heart is frequently involved in hemochromatosis with brownish discoloration of the myocardium; diffuse, severe involvement results in a soft, brown, dilated organ with marked dilatation of the right ventricle and vena cava. Hemosiderin granules in myocardial fibers and myocardial fibrosis are evident. Heart failure may occur or arrhythmias due to hemosiderin in conduction system fibers. Rickettsial diseases are frequently complicated by myocarditis, especially in scrub typhus and in about 50 percent of cases of epidemic typhus and Rocky Mountain spotted fever. Rickettsiae cause a systemic vasculitis that forms the basis for the interstitial myocarditis and other lesions. Sarcoidosis is now recognized as a cause of heart disease, even without the existence of cor pulmonale. Formation of sarcoid granulomas may be accompanied by considerable fibrosis, myocardial damage, heart failure, and sudden death. More often, cor pulmonale results from extensive lung involvement. Metastatic malignancy is the most common tumor to involve the heart, especially the pericardium, by vascular dissemination or direct extension. The primary tumor is most frequently carcinoma of lung or breast, lymphoma, leukemia, or malignant melanoma. Tumor involvement of pericardium frequently causes hemorrhagic effusion.

202. The answer is D (4). *(Anderson, ed 9. pp 650-652, 675.)* Ankylosing spondylitis, also known as Marie-Strümpell disease, was previously classified under the rheumatoid disorders, especially rheumatoid spondylitis, but evidence shows that it is separate from rheumatoid disease. Ankylosing spondylitis has a high incidence in men, whereas rheumatoid arthritis occurs predominantly in women. It is negative for rheumatoid factor in the sera and, other than involving the vertebrae, usually spares the peripheral joints. Rheumatic myocarditis is characterized by Aschoff cells in interstitial myocardium, which are not seen in the cardiac lesions of ankylosing spondylitis. Ankylosing spondylitis most closely resembles syphilitic aortic valvulitis and aortitis in that the aortic valve ring is dilated, with thickened, rolled aortic valve leaflets and adhesions that cause fusion of the commissure. The tunica media of the aorta frequently shows necrosis and a lymphocytic infiltration as in syphilis. Rheumatoid heart disease, on the other hand, shows granulomatous lesions resembling the rheumatoid nodules seen in the skin and in soft tissues over the joints.

203-206. The answers are: 203-A, 204-C, 205-A, 206-E. *(Robbins, ed 4. pp 643-648.)* The cardiomyopathies (CMP) may be classified into primary and secondary forms. The primary forms are mainly idiopathic (unknown cause). The causes of secondary CMP are many and range from alcoholism (probably the most common cause in the United States) to metabolic disorders to toxins and poisons. Whereas there are not many gross organ and microscopic anatomical features of CMP, a few rather characteristic hallmarks are well recognized in separating the types. However, extensive clinical, historical, and laboratory data contribute as much if not more to classification of the type of CMP present than does biopsy or even the postmortem heart examination.

Hypertrophic CMP encompasses those cases in which the major gross abnormality is to be found within the interventricular septum, which is usually thicker than the left ventricle. If there is obstruction of the ventricular outflow tract, there will be moderate hypertrophy in the left ventricles as well, but the septum usually remains thicker, yielding an appearance of asymmetric hypertrophy. This form of CMP occurs in families (rarely sporadically) and is thought to be autosomal dominant. Up to one-third of these patients have been known to die sudden cardiac deaths, often under conditions of physical exertion. Histologically, the myofibers interconnect at angles and are hypertrophied.

In dilated (congestive) CMP, the ventricular chambers are markedly dilated, with the walls either of normal thickness or thinner than normal. Whereas many idiopathic cases exist, some patients have a history of heavy alcohol intake. The microscopic appearance is not distinctive. The ventricles may have mural thrombi.

Constrictive (restrictive) CMP is associated in the United States with amyloidosis and endocardial fibroelastosis and is so named because the infiltration and deposition of amyloid in the endomyocardium and the layering of collagen and elastin over the endocardium affect the ability of the ventricles to accommodate blood volume during asystole. The heart is more likely to be so involved if the systemic amyloidosis is associated with primary systemic or plasma cell tumors (myeloma). Endocardial fibroelastosis occurs mainly in infants and in the first 1 to 2 years of life and causes a prominent fibroelastic covering to form over the endocardium of the left ventricle. There may be associated aortic coarctation, ventricular septal defects, mitral valve defects, and other abnormalities.

Endomyocardial fibrosis is a form of restrictive CMP found mainly in young adults and children in Southeast Asia and Africa, where it accounts for a not insignificant number of deaths in these age groups. It differs from endocardial fibroelastosis in the United States in that elastic fibers are not present. Its cause is totally unknown.

207-210. The answers are: 207-A, 208-C, 209-D, 210-B. (*Anderson, ed 9. pp 650-652, 659-661, 778-780.*) Primary myocarditis, an isolated lesion that is not secondary to a generalized disease, is most commonly caused by such agents as type B coxsackievirus, echoviruses, and *Toxoplasma gondii*.

Streptococci are generally considered the causative agents of rheumatic fever; and although group A β-hemolytic streptococci are most strongly implicated, viruses continue to be suspected as among the causes of this systemic nonsuppurative inflammatory disease. Abundant evidence supports the view that antibodies generated in the immunologic reaction to infection with group A β-hemolytic streptococcus cross-react with myocardial fibers, smooth muscle cells, and connective tissue glycoproteins. Aschoff bodies, produced in response to this cross-reaction, are regarded as pathognomonic for rheumatic fever.

Aortic aneurysms of luetic carditis constitute the tertiary manifestation of syphilis and become evident 15 to 20 years after persons have contracted infection with *Treponema pallidum*. Elastic tissue and smooth muscle cells of the media undergo ischemic destruction as a result of the treponemal infection. As a consequence of ischemia in the media, musculoelastic support is lost, leading to aortic aneurysms, widening of the aortic valve ring, and narrowing of the coronary ostia.

Suppurative pericarditis is a form of acute pericarditis that can be caused by *Mycobacterium tuberculosis* and is considered to invariably denote entry into the pericardium of bacterial, mycotic, or parasitic agents. In the suppurative pericarditis caused by *M. tuberculosis* (tuberculous pericarditis), tuberculosis of the mediastinal nodes has been a finding in the majority of affected adults. Up to 500 ml of thick fluid (typical of caseation necrosis) containing granulocytes, erythrocytes, and, in 50 percent of patients who have tuberculous pericarditis, tubercle bacilli may be found in the pericardium.

211-214. The answers are: 211-D, 212-A, 213-B, 214-E. *(Anderson, ed 9. pp 774-775. Robbins, ed 4. pp 155-157, 576-579, 1020-1021.)* Berry aneurysms in the circle of Willis have been noted in about one-sixth of patients with adult polycystic renal disease. Subarachnoid hemorrhage from these, because of hypertension, accounts for death in about 10 percent of patients with adult polycystic renal disease.

Ehlers-Danlos syndromes (EDSs) are a group of eight syndromes characterized by defects in collagen synthesis. In EDS IV there is deficient synthesis of type III collagen and a tendency to rupture of muscular arteries, including dissecting aneurysms of the aorta. A high incidence of dissecting aneurysm also occurs in Marfan's syndrome and it may occur in coarctation of the aorta.

Both Takayasu's and Kawasaki's diseases (mucocutaneous lymph node syndrome) are examples of arteritis. Kawasaki's disease is thought to be an immune complex disorder, possibly caused by *Propionibacterium acnes,* although a retrovirus has been suggested. It was first recognized in Japan, but there have been several outbreaks in the continental U.S. and in Hawaii. A skin rash, lymphadenopathy, arthritis, and arteritis are predominant. Coronary arteritis results in aneurysms and is associated with myocarditis and sometimes infarction. The disease characteristically affects boys under 4 years old.

Takayasu's arteritis, or "pulseless disease," is most common in young women and affects large and medium arteries, especially the aorta and its larger branches. Aneurysms are common in the abdominal and distal thoracic aorta, especially in older patients. There may be thrombosis of vessels arising from the aortic arch and many cases demonstrate the aortic arch syndrome. Marked weakening of the pulses in the upper extremities is noted. This arteritis has been known as *aortic arch syndrome, primary aortitis,* and *giant-cell arteritis of the aorta,* in addition to other synonyms. Arteriosclerotic aneurysms are also common in the abdominal aorta; syphilitic aneurysm is practically limited to the thoracic segment.

215-217. The answers are: 215-D, 216-C, 217-E. *(Anderson, ed 9. pp 685, 688.)* Cardiac manifestations in some patients with the carcinoid syndrome are the result of fibrosis of the tricuspid and pulmonary valve cusps. Fibrous plaques form usually on the right ventricular endocardium and valve leaflets, resulting in tricuspid insufficiency and pulmonic stenosis, possibly under the influence of 5-hydroxytryptamine from the carcinoid tumor.

Cardiac enlargement is seen in myxedema with a pale, flabby, dilated heart; marked interstitial edema; and myocardial basophilic degeneration. The cardiac enlargement in thiamine (vitamin B_1) deficiency involves a characteristic globose shape from concurrent dilatation of the chamber and ventricular hypertrophy. In the United States, beriberi heart is usually a result of chronic alcoholism.

Fatty degeneration of the heart must be separated from fatty infiltration (usually in the right ventricle), which occurs in obesity. Fatty degeneration characteristic of severe anemia affects the subendocardial myocardium, particularly in the left ventricle. Lipid vacuoles in the myocardial fibers appear grossly as irregular, yellowish streaks or lines of involved muscle, alternating with lines of unaffected muscle, and giving a "tigroid," "tabby cat," or "thrush-breast" appearance. Fatty degeneration is seen with anoxia, toxins, sepsis, and neonatal deaths.

Respiratory System

DIRECTIONS: Each question below contains five suggested responses. Select the **one best** response to each question.

218. Horner's syndrome is associated with

(A) lymphangitis carcinomatosa
(B) bronchial carcinoid
(C) exophthalmos
(D) tumor of the superior sulcus
(E) thoracocervical venous dilatation

219. Alpha$_1$-antitrypsin deficiency is associated with

(A) thalassemia
(B) nephrotic syndrome
(C) panlobular emphysema
(D) centrilobular emphysema
(E) anthracosis

220. Human infection caused by the dog heartworm, *Dirofilaria immitis,* may cause

(A) bronchitis
(B) subcutaneous nodules
(C) thoracic lymphadenopathy
(D) conjunctival infection
(E) pulmonary infarction

221. A young woman succumbed after an 8-month course of severe dyspnea, fatigue, and cyanosis that followed an uneventful delivery of a healthy infant. At necropsy, small atheromas were present in the large and small branches of the pulmonary arteries. Which of the following findings can be predicted in the histologic slides of the lungs?

(A) Diffuse hemorrhage and infarctions
(B) Diffuse alveolar hyaline membranes
(C) Severe atelectasis and edema
(D) Marked medial hypertrophy of pulmonary arterioles
(E) Multiple pulmonary emboli

222. Which of the following bronchogenic carcinomas is associated with production of parathormone-like substances?

(A) Bronchioloalveolar carcinoma
(B) Papillary adenocarcinoma
(C) Acinar adenocarcinoma
(D) Squamous cell carcinoma
(E) Oat cell carcinoma

223. The cells in the photomicrograph below appeared in a cytologic specimen of sputum from a 52-year-old man with chest pain, some loss of weight, and a nonproductive cough of 8 months' duration. Which of the following is the most likely diagnosis?

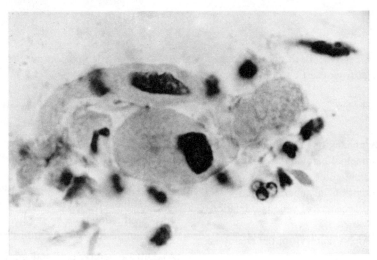

(A) Oat cell (small-cell undifferentiated) carcinoma
(B) Adenocarcinoma
(C) Pneumocystis pneumonia
(D) Squamous metaplasia
(E) Squamous cell carcinoma

---

224. A patient hospitalized for fractures of the long bones who develops mental dysfunction, increasing respiratory insufficiency, and renal failure should be suspected of having

(A) fat embolism syndrome
(B) disseminated intravascular coagulopathy
(C) myocardial infarction
(D) aortic valve disease
(E) respiratory distress syndrome

225. The major pathologic injury in interstitial lung disease is generally accepted to be

(A) bronchopneumonia
(B) bronchiolitis
(C) alveolitis
(D) bronchitis
(E) diffuse pneumonia

226. A 48-year-old woman with a 26 pack-year history of cigarette smoking was noted to have abnormal cells (malignancy is suspected) in sputum cytology. The chest x-ray is presented (right). What is the most likely diagnosis?

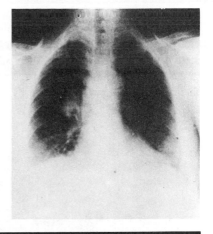

(A) Sarcoidosis
(B) Adenocarcinoma
(C) Breast carcinoma
(D) Small-cell carcinoma
(E) Squamous cell carcinoma

227. The organism that is most likely to cause the necrotizing pulmonary lesion shown in the photomicrograph below is

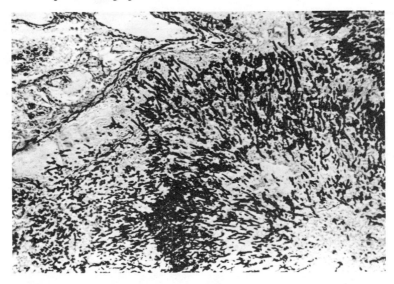

(A) *Pseudomonas aeruginosa*
(B) *Mycobacterium tuberculosis*
(C) *Pneumocystis carinii*
(D) *Trichinella spiralis*
(E) *Candida albicans*

228. Acute lymphoblastic leukemia was diagnosed in a 10-year-old child. When this child later developed a patchy pulmonary infiltrate and respiratory insufficiency, a lung biopsy was performed. The material obtained by biopsy was then stained with Gomori's methenamine-silver stain and is shown in the photomicrograph below. In consideration of the patient's signs and microscopic evaluations, the prognosis is now complicated by

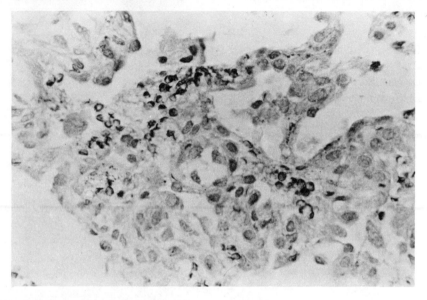

(A) *Pseudomonas* pneumonia
(B) *Aspergillus* pneumonia
(C) *Pneumocystis carinii* pneumonia
(D) pneumococcal pneumonia
(E) influenza pneumonia

DIRECTIONS: Each question below contains four suggested responses of which **one or more** is correct. Select

A	if	**1, 2, and 3**	are correct
B	if	**1 and 3**	are correct
C	if	**2 and 4**	are correct
D	if	**4**	is correct
E	if	**1, 2, 3, and 4**	are correct

229. Legionnaires' disease is suspected in an adult hospital maintenance worker who became ill with headaches, malaise, and a dry cough. The diagnosis can be confirmed rapidly and reliably by

(1) open lung biopsy
(2) chest roentgenography
(3) checking serum agglutinin levels
(4) immunofluorescence testing

230. Molecular biology of lung tumors has shown that

(1) K-*ras* oncogenes are activated in many adenocarcinomas
(2) epidermoid cancers express high levels of receptor for transforming growth factor
(3) small-cell carcinomas show a deletion in the short arm of chromosome 3
(4) abnormal retinoblastoma antioncogenes are common in adenocarcinoma

231. Common tumors or cysts in the superior mediastinum include

(1) metastatic carcinoma
(2) bronchogenic cyst
(3) thymoma
(4) neurogenic tumors

232. In AIDS patients, evidence that hypoimmunity exists comes from the

(1) lack of intracellular antimicrobial activity of macrophages
(2) absence or abnormality of macrophage activation
(3) absence of B cells, especially plasma cells
(4) impaired production of lymphokines

233. "Usual interstitial pneumonia" (fibrosing alveolitis) is characterized by

(1) pulmonary insufficiency and death occurring within a year of the onset of symptoms
(2) cellular thickening of alveolar walls with fibrosis and chronic inflammatory infiltrates
(3) an increased incidence of primary pulmonary malignancy
(4) alveolar-capillary block

SUMMARY OF DIRECTIONS

A	B	C	D	E
1, 2, 3 only	1, 3 only	2, 4 only	4 only	All are correct

234. The condition seen below in the gross photograph of a sagittal section of the lung may occur in which of the following?

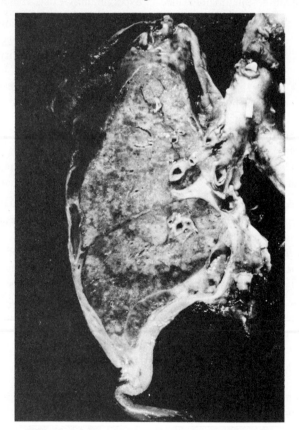

(1) Adenocarcinoma
(2) Oat cell carcinoma
(3) Malignant mesothelioma
(4) Benign spindle cell mesothelioma

235. The photomicrograph of the bronchial washing specimen shown below depicts

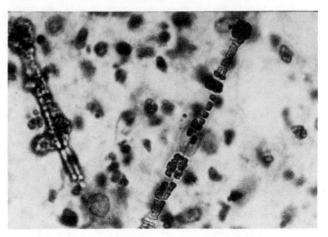

(1) Schaumann bodies
(2) ferruginous bodies
(3) cholesterol crystals
(4) asbestos bodies

SUMMARY OF DIRECTIONS

A	B	C	D	E
1, 2, 3 only	1, 3 only	2, 4 only	4 only	All are correct

Questions 236-237

Shown in the photomicrograph below is a section of alveolar tissue that was taken at autopsy of a 4-day-old premature infant.

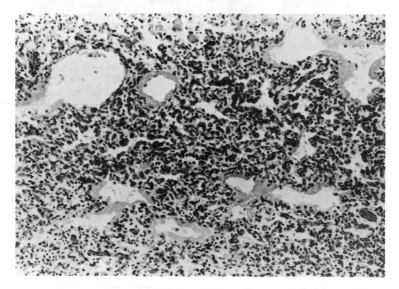

236. The pathologic process that is evident is consistent with

(1) congenital pulmonary cystic malformation
(2) extralobar pulmonary sequestration
(3) primary fungal pneumonitis
(4) respiratory distress syndrome (hyaline membrane disease)

237. A similar histopathologic condition can be seen in lungs of adults who have

(1) viral pneumonia
(2) uremia
(3) pulmonary irradiation
(4) severe bacterial infection

238. A 40-year-old woman undergoes excision of a well-circumscribed lesion in the subpleural upper lung after a shadow was seen on a preemployment chest x-ray. The lesion is demonstrated in the photomicrograph below. Which of the following statements applies to this disease process?

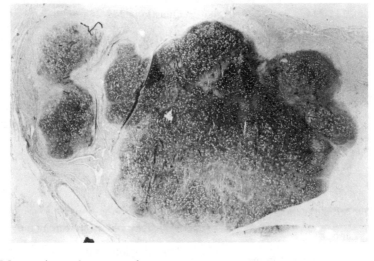

(1) Metastasis can be expected
(2) This is a relatively rare tumor
(3) The tumor is radiosensitive
(4) The tumor is diagnosed predominantly in adults

239. Extrapulmonary manifestations of bronchogenic carcinoma

(1) include Cushing's syndrome
(2) include inappropriate antidiuretic hormone activity
(3) include peripheral neuropathy and myopathy
(4) occur in patients who have normal bone scans

240. A 2-year-old infant seen in the emergency room with respiratory distress, fever, dyspnea, wheezing, and sternal retractions would probably have which of the following in terminal episodes?

(1) Apparently normal appearance in gross examination
(2) Marked pleural effusions
(3) Bronchiolar inflammatory infiltrates
(4) Hyaline membranes

DIRECTIONS: Each group of questions below consists of lettered headings followed by a set of numbered items. For each numbered item select the **one** lettered heading with which it is **most** closely associated. Each lettered heading may be used **once, more than once, or not at all.**

Questions 241-244

Match the most characteristic finding with each respiratory disorder.

(A) Myasthenic syndrome
(B) Fungal infection
(C) Hemorrhagic interstitial pneumonitis
(D) Nasal mucosal ulcerations
(E) Asthmatic bronchitis

241. Wegener's granulomatosis

242. Oat cell carcinoma

243. Byssinosis

244. Goodpasture's syndrome

Questions 245-248

For each tumor, choose its most common site of origin.

(A) Nasal cavity
(B) Neuroendocrine cells of bronchi
(C) Submucosal bronchial glands
(D) Terminal bronchioles
(E) Bronchial blood vessels

245. Bronchial carcinoid

246. Bronchioloalveolar carcinoma

247. Adenoid cystic carcinoma

248. Angiofibroma

Respiratory System
Answers

218. The answer is D. *(Robbins, ed 4. pp 801-804.)* Horner's syndrome occurs with apical (superior sulcus) tumors of any type (Pancoast tumor). The syndrome is characterized by enophthalmos, ptosis, miosis, and anhidrosis on the same side as the lesion due to invasion of the cervical sympathetic. Involvement of the brachial plexus causes pain and paralysis in the ulnar nerve distribution. Venous dilatation of the upper thorax and neck is seen in the superior vena caval syndrome because of compression or invasion by lung cancer or lymphoma. Lymphangitic carcinomatosis usually results from spread of metastatic tumors within subpleural lymphatics.

219. The answer is C. *(Robbins, ed 4. pp 137, 159, 767-770.)* Patients who are homozygous for alpha$_1$-antitrypsin deficiency develop severe panlobular emphysema, often before the age of 40. This genetic disorder accounts for about 10 percent of cases of emphysema. Other factors in the pathogenesis of emphysema include air pollution and smoking. The disorder results from any variant of the numerous alleles on the chromosomal locus of Pi (proteinase inhibitor). Cigarette smoking greatly accelerates the emphysema in the homozygous (Pi ZZ) state.

220. The answer is E. *(Robbins, ed 4. pp 419-420.)* Pulmonary dirofilariasis is caused by a single larva of the dog heartworm, *D. immitis,* which embolizes from the right heart to a peripheral pulmonary artery and causes a small infarct. This nodular or "coin" lesion may be mistaken for a tumor. Histologically, granulomatous or mixed inflammation borders infarcted lung with a central dead, or degenerate, larva. The lesion should be excluded when a necrotic lung nodule is found at surgery, but multiple sections may be needed to find the larva. Animal filariae such as *D. immitis* or *D. tenuis* (which usually infects raccoons) are arthropod-borne. *D. tenuis* may cause conjunctival and skin infections including subcutaneous nodules. North American *Brugia* (which generally infects raccoons and lynx) involves lymphatics and causes enlargement of one cervical/thoracic lymph node.

221. The answer is D. *(Robbins, ed 4. pp 764-765.)* Many pathologic pulmonary changes can be found in the lungs of patients who expire under conditions of progressive, unexplained dyspnea, fatigue, and cyanosis. These changes range from pulmonary fibrosis to hypersensitivity pneumonitis and to recurrent, multiple pulmonary emboli. Furthermore, traditional hospital treatment modalities for progressive pulmonary deterioration (including high oxygen delivery, overhydration, lack of pulmonary ventilation, irregular ventilation by mechanical respiratory assist [PEEP], and superimposed nosocomially acquired pneumonitis) can complicate pulmonary pathologic findings. However, unremitting, progressive dyspnea, cyanosis, and fatigue in a young woman should suggest the diagnosis of primary pulmonary hypertension. Pulmonary vascular sclerosis is always associated with pulmonary hypertension primary or secondary to other states, such as emphysema and mitral stenosis.

222. The answer is D. *(Robbins, ed 4. pp 294-296, 801.)* Squamous cell carcinoma, the most frequent type of bronchogenic carcinoma (25 to 30 percent), is the type most often associated with hypercalcemia. The hypercalcemia may be related to osteolytic bone metastases, but hypercalcemia as a paraneoplastic syndrome may occur in the absence of skeletal metastases. This form of hypercalcemia is caused by tumor production of parathormone-like substances, or prostaglandin E, or other calcium-mobilizing tumor products such as growth factors involved in the histogenesis of the tumor. These probably bind to the parathyroid hormone receptors in bone to mimic the calcium-mobilizing action of parathormone. Hypercalcemia is rare with oat cell tumors, which are much more likely to produce ACTH-like (Cushing's syndrome) or ADH-like substances.

223. The answer is E. *(Takahashi, ed 2. pp 305-306.)* The cells shown have rather bizarre shape, marked nuclear hyperchromasia and irregularity, an increase in nuclear area and in nucleocytoplasmic ratio, and marked variation in cell size and shape — all criteria suggestive of malignancy. Malignant cells of this type (often with orangeophilic cytoplasm) found in sputum are diagnostic of squamous cell carcinoma. In adenocarcinoma the cells form clusters and have less hyperchromatic nuclei, but prominent nucleoli, and vacuolated cytoplasm. Oat cell carcinoma has much smaller cells and tight clusters with nuclear molding. *Pneumocystis* is seen as a very fine, bubbly or frothy (pink) organism in sputum.

224. The answer is A. *(Robbins, ed 4. pp 110-111.)* Fat embolism syndrome can supervene as a complication within 3 days following severe trauma to the long bones. However, the pathogenesis must be regarded as unknown because simple entrance of microglobular fat into the circulation as a result of damage to small vessels in marrow tissue occurs in over 90 percent of patients with trauma and bone fracture, yet the syndrome occurs in only a minority of such patients. Laboratory and clinical findings can simulate those of intravascular coagulopathy, which may be a component of fat embolism syndrome, with a major difference of split products of fibrin seen mainly in intravascular coagulopathy. Plasma levels of free fatty acids are elevated in fat embolism and may contribute to pulmonary vascular alterations. At autopsy fat material can be demonstrated in fat stains of frozen sections of lung, brain, and kidney in patients who had the syndrome.

225. The answer is C. *(Robbins, ed 4. pp 789-791.)* In diffuse interstitial lung disease (ILD) the early and major event is damage to the alveolar walls. First, an interstitial inflammation affects mainly the septae (interstitial alveolitis) with edema of the alveolar walls and an infiltrate of lymphocytes and monocyte-macrophages. The alveolar lining cells (mostly type I) are injured or become necrotic and are replaced by proliferating type II cells creating a cuboidal epithelial lining; alveolar endothelial cells are also injured, allowing exudation of fluid into the interstitium. If reversal does not occur, the changes become chronic with eventual fibrous scarring of alveolar walls, impaired respiratory function, and pulmonary hypertension. Causes of ILD include occupational exposure to inorganic dust (asbestos, silica), gases, aerosols, and organic dust, in addition to drugs (bleomycin, busulfan, nitrofurantoin) and infections (cytomegalovirus and tuberculosis). The major interstitial lung diseases of unknown cause include sarcoidosis and idiopathic pulmonary fibrosis (Hamman-Rich syndrome).

226. The answer is D. *(Anderson, ed 9. pp 1011-1013.)* The chest x-ray in this clinical example demonstrates a central mass in the region of the hilum of the right lung. The differential diagnosis of a radiographic central mass includes consideration of undifferentiated small-cell carcinoma, sarcoidosis, lymphoma, and, less commonly, other forms of bronchogenic carcinoma. In sputum cytology, small-cell carcinomas demonstrate clusters of lymphocyte-like tumor cells in strands, with adjacent tumor nuclei indentation (nuclear molding). The incidence of carcinoma of the lung in males is dropping somewhat, but the overall incidence continues because of greater numbers of women taking up the cigarette habit in recent years, with many of these women starting in their teens. As a consequence, small-cell (oat cell) carcinoma is being seen with greater frequency in women.

227. The answer is E. *(Anderson, ed 9. pp 411-413.)* Gomori's methenamine-silver staining technique emphasizes the pseudohyphae and yeast forms of *Candida* species. The pattern of vessel invasion is characteristic of many pathogenic fungi, including *Candida*. Such infections tend to occur in immunologically suppressed patients with other severe, usually neoplastic, diseases.

228. The answer is C. *(Anderson, ed 9. p 948.)* Infection by the protozoan *Pneumocystis carinii* is characterized by the presence of oval and helmet-shaped organisms whose capsules are made more visible by use of Gomori's methenamine-silver staining technique. This organism, although having low virulence, is opportunistic, for it is often seen to attack severely ill, immunologically depressed patients.

229. The answer is D (4). *(Robbins, ed 4. pp 347-348. Stout, N Engl J Med 306: 466, 1982.)* Since the widely publicized outbreak of Legionnaires' disease at an American Legion convention in Philadelphia in 1976, Legionnaires' bacillus (*Legionella pneumophila*) has been isolated in various buildings and institutions, especially in air ventilation systems, air conditioners, and even in tap water, faucets, and shower heads in a large hospital. The organism responsible is a gram-negative bacillus that is difficult to isolate and stain in tissues and that causes a patchy alveolar space infiltration of polymorphonuclear leukocytes, scattered round cells, and histiocytes. Silver stains may be used to identify the bacilli within inflammatory cells. It is possible but not expeditious to gain supporting clinical evidence that the organism is responsible for pneumonitis by such means as lung biopsy and serum agglutination, but tracheal aspirates may contain this rare organism, which can be identified relatively rapidly via direct immunofluorescence in the laboratories of large hospitals. Successful termination of the infection has been achieved with erythromycin and tetracycline.

230. The answer is A (1, 2, 3). *(Anderson, ed 9. pp 603, 1015.)* Epidermoid carcinomas express high levels of receptor for transforming growth factor (alpha and epidermal GF). This receptor has tyrosine kinase activity and may be permanently attuned to growth or may fail to respond to normal controls. It is produced by the c-*erbB* oncogene. Abnormalities of retinoblastoma antioncogenes are common in small-cell carcinoma and atypical carcinoid. Several chromosomal deletions are common in small-cell cancer, but the short-arm deletion in chromosome 3 is paramount, while amplification of c-*myc* oncogene is associated with very aggressive behavior. Activation of the K-*ras* oncogene may play a role in pathogenesis of adenocarcinoma of the lung.

231. The answer is B (1, 3). *(Robbins, ed 4. pp 803-804.)* The superior mediastinum consists of structures cephalad to the pericardial reflection of the heart. Metastatic carcinoma is fairly frequent in the superior mediastinum, arising often from lung or breast primaries, and less frequently from testis or kidney. Bronchogenic and pericardial cysts occur in the middle mediastinum, whereas neurogenic tumors such as neurofibroma and schwannoma are in the posterior mediastinum. Thymoma is found in the anterosuperior mediastinum. Lymphoma, especially Hodgkin's disease, is common in all mediastinal compartments and involves paratracheal lymph nodes in the superior mediastinum. Seminoma and metastatic choriocarcinoma from the testis are not uncommon. Parathyroid tumors and thyroid lesions occupy both the superior and anterior mediastinum. Retrosternal extension of a goiter, presenting as a superior mediastinal mass, is not unusual.

232. The answer is C (2, 4). *(Murray, N Engl J Med 310:883, 1984.)* Recent work has shown that a markedly reduced and even absent production of lymphokines occurs in AIDS patients. T lymphocytes from AIDS patients have a reduced capacity to produce gamma interferon even in response to microbial antigen. In in vitro experiments, if normal lymphokines or gamma interferon is added to monocytes from AIDS patients, there is effective activity against intracellular microorganisms. B cells, including plasma cells, are not ordinarily decreased in AIDS patients, especially during the early phases of the disease, and may even be seen in increased numbers within the lymph nodes, as the helper T cells are reduced. Opportunistic infections in AIDS patients may result from reduced gamma interferon and other lymphokine production.

233. The answer is C (2, 4). *(Anderson, ed 9. p 971.)* The morphologic features of usual interstitial pneumonia (UIP) include interstitial edema and edema with hyaline membrane formation within the small air spaces in early lesions. An infiltrate of monocytes and lymphocytes then occurs. Regenerating alveolar epithelium relines damaged alveoli by "growing over" the alveolar exudate and thus incorporates this material into the interstitium. Fibrosis follows and may produce a pattern of randomly communicating air spaces lined by fibrous walls and metaplastic epithelium referred to as "honeycomb lung." Many people with UIP survive for many years. No increase in the incidence of primary malignancy has been described.

234. The answer is B (1, 3). *(Robbins, ed 4. pp 800, 806-808.)* Malignant mesothelioma and adenocarcinoma are two neoplasms that may involve the pleural surfaces as seen in the gross photograph. Malignant mesothelioma arises from the pleural surfaces and is thus a pleural neoplasm developing in association with significant and chronic exposure to asbestos, usually occupationally incurred. As the malignant mesothelioma spreads, it lines the pleural surfaces including the fissures through the lobes of the lungs and results in a tight and constricting encasement. This restricts the excursions of the lungs during ventilation. Adenocarcinoma of the lung also may invade the pleural surfaces and spread in an advancing manner throughout the pleural lining surfaces. The differential diagnosis histologically between an epithelial type of malignant mesothelioma and an adenocarcinoma may be difficult and sometimes impossible without special techniques. Oat cell carcinoma usually arises in the central portions of the lungs near the hilum and does not invade the pleura in a spreading fashion. Benign spindle (fibrous) mesothelioma of the lung arises as a discrete mass that is spherical to ovoid in shape in a subpleural configuration and expands as this localized mass without spread over the surfaces.

235. The answer is C (2, 4). *(Anderson, ed 9. pp 235, 587, 1003.)* The segmented or beaded, often dumbbell-shaped bodies are ferruginous bodies that are probably asbestos fibers coated with iron and protein. The term ferruginous body is applied to other inhaled fibers that become iron coated; however, in a patient with interstitial lung fibrosis or pleural plaques, ferruginous bodies are probably asbestos bodies. The type of asbestos mainly used in America is chrysotile, mined in Canada, and it is much less likely to cause mesothelioma or lung cancer than is crocidolite (blue asbestos), which has limited use and is mined in South Africa. Cigarette smoking potentiates the relatively mild carcinogenic effect of asbestos. Laminated spherical (Schaumann) bodies are found in granulomas of sarcoid and chronic berylliosis.

236. The answer is D (4). *(Anderson, ed 9. pp 838-839.)* The photomicrograph shows classic hyaline membranes coating alveolar sacs and ducts and is diagnostic of the respiratory distress syndrome of the newborn. The eosinophilic, fibrin-like material is related to the alveolar surfactants. Atelectasis is usually also present, especially in premature infants. The deposited material appears not to form in utero, as it is found in infants who have breathed and is not found in stillborns. There is a direct correlation, however, between severity and the degree of prematurity.

237. The answer is E (all). *(Anderson, ed 9. pp 925-926.)* The presence of hyaline membranes indicates a diagnosis of acute alveolar injury, which can occur in all the conditions mentioned. Indeed, the alveoli-lining, fibrin-like material may be found in multiple conditions of circulatory compromise and in poor perfusion states, such as hypovolemia; it may also be seen where 100% oxygen has been used for longer than 32 hours (e.g., "shock lung" of Vietnam casualties). At autopsy, the lungs are relatively airless and heavy, and this finding is frequently accompanied by pulmonary edema and hemorrhage.

238. The answer is C (2, 4). *(Robbins, ed 4. p 803.)* Pulmonary hamartomas are not common tumors, but it is very important to recognize them radiologically as well as pathologically because simple, conservative excision is curative. The lesion is composed of components of tissue normally found in the region where it develops, but in abnormal amounts and configurations. This is the definition of hamartomas in general. In the lung, they are composed of hyaline cartilage, variable smooth muscle, and respiratory epithelium-lined clefts. Minimal growth has been recorded with chest x-rays, but rapid growth (as seen in lung carcinoma) would be an unusual event for pulmonary hamartomas. They are never necrotic with cavity or air-fluid level formation. Pulmonary hamartomas have a peak incidence at age 60.

239. The answer is E (all). *(Anderson, ed 9. p 1013.)* All the systemic symptoms and syndromes mentioned occur in conjunction with bronchogenic carcinomas of various histologic types. The most common endocrine manifestation is probably Cushing's syndrome, but the number and variety of tumor-associated endocrine syndromes have increased dramatically in recent years. Additional neuromuscular abnormalities associated with lung tumors include mental status changes ranging from impaired acuity to dementia, degenerative myopathy, and a myasthenia gravis–like syndrome. Hypercalcemia may be seen in patients with squamous carcinoma and large-cell carcinoma who have no evidence of bony metastases, but it is not seen in patients with oat cell carcinoma.

240. The answer is B (1, 3). *(Anderson, ed 9. pp 930-932.)* The presentation of an infant of 2 years or less with acute respiratory distress syndrome manifested clinically by sternal retractions, fever, and rapid breathing suggests bronchiolitis. Infants who die of upper respiratory infections usually have pneumonia or bronchiolitis, and the causes most often involve respiratory syncytial virus, followed in frequency by parainfluenza virus, adenovirus, and *Mycoplasma pneumoniae*. These organisms can cause bronchiolitis, which is manifested pathologically by infiltration of inflammatory cells of the peribronchial tissues as well as the lumens and walls of the small airways. This will produce pinpoint narrowing of the small airways, which may or may not be seen at autopsy. Often the lungs will appear normal at autopsy unless close examination is done of the small airways.

241-244. The answers are: 241-D, 242-A, 243-E, 244-C. *(Anderson, ed 9. p 1013. Robbins, ed 4. pp 574, 794.)* Oat cell carcinomas, which are of neuroendocrine origin and display neurosecretory granules on electron microscopy, may cause a variety of syndromes, some from direct synthesis of hormones such as ACTH and serotonin. Other effects, not well understood, on the neuromuscular system include central encephalopathy and Eaton-Lambert syndrome, a myasthenic syndrome resulting from impaired release of acetylcholine and usually associated with pulmonary oat cell carcinoma. Oat cell carcinomas form 20 to 25 percent of primary lung tumors, occur most frequently in middle-aged or older men, have a strong association with cigarette smoking, and carry a poor prognosis.

Both Wegener's granulomatosis, a syndrome of necrotizing vasculitis with necrotizing granulomas of nasopharynx and lung, and Goodpasture's syndrome, a disease produced by autoantibodies directed against basement membranes, typically involve both the lung and kidney. Goodpasture's syndrome is characterized by development of a necrotizing hemorrhagic interstitial pneumonitis and rapidly progressing glomerulonephritis because of antibodies directed against the capillary basement membrane in alveolar septae and glomeruli. Prognosis for Goodpasture's syndrome has been markedly improved by intensive plasma exchange to remove circulating antibasement membrane antibodies and immunosuppressive therapy to inhibit further antibody production. In Wegener's granulomatosis, the nose, sinus, antrum, and trachea often exhibit ulcerations. Originally lethal, prognosis is now much improved by immunosuppressive drugs.

Byssinosis, which is caused by inhalation of cotton, flax, or hemp dust, takes the form of an asthmatic bronchitis, rather than involving distal lung structures, as with other organic dusts that cause extrinsic allergic alveolitis. Prolonged exposure causes chronic lung disease with chronic bronchitis, emphysema, and interstitial granulomas.

245-248. The answers are: 245-B, 246-D, 247-C, 248-A. *(Anderson, ed 9. p 1017. Robbins, ed 4. pp 800, 802-803, 814-815.)* Bronchial carcinoids form about 5 percent of lung tumors. Sex incidence is equal and many patients are under 40 years of age. No relation to cigarette smoking or environmental factors is known. The origin is the neuroendocrine argentaffin cells of bronchial mucosa (Kultschitzsky cells). The carcinoid syndrome (diarrhea, facial flushing, and cyanosis) rarely occurs in disease confined to the lung. Carcinoid belongs to the group of amine precursor uptake and decarboxylation (APUD) tumors.

Bronchioloalveolar carcinoma, a form of adenocarcinoma, arises from terminal bronchioles and extends to line alveolar spaces throughout peripheral lung tissue, often causing a pneumonia-like picture grossly and radiologically. Ultrastructurally it consists of mucin-secreting bronchiolar cells, Clara cells, and, rarely, type II pneumocytes.

Adenoid cystic carcinoma may arise at any level of the respiratory tract where there are mucous glands and is the most common tumor in the upper third of the trachea. Histopathologic appearance is similar to adenoid cystic carcinoma of minor salivary glands with a cribriform, lace-like pattern of either duct-lining secretory cells or myoepithelial cells. Pools of mucoid material are actually extracellular matrix.

Nasopharyngeal angiofibroma is a highly vascular tumor that can cause heavy bleeding and occurs in young males. Other rare, but distinctive nasal tumors include isolated plasmacytoma, lymphoepithelioma, olfactory neuroblastoma (esthesioneuroblastoma), inverted papilloma, and carcinomas of epidermoid and transitional cell types.

Gastrointestinal System

DIRECTIONS: Each question below contains five suggested responses. Select the **one best** response to each question.

249. The photomicrograph below shows the colonic wall 30 cm from the anal margin in a man with severe bloody diarrhea. All the statements regarding this condition are true EXCEPT

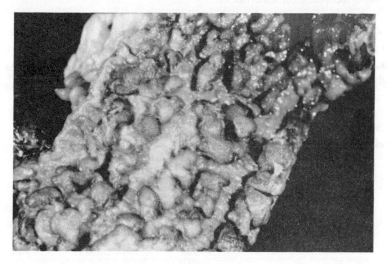

(A) inflammation is usually limited to the lamina propria
(B) multiple crypt abscesses are commonly seen
(C) atypical cytologic changes occur in the mucosa
(D) granulomas occur in the mucosa
(E) endarteritis obliterans occurs in the submucosal arteries

250. A 25-year-old schoolteacher was well until she attended a church bazaar where she partook copiously of barbecued turkey. The following day she developed bloody diarrhea, crampy pain, and tenesmus. A gastroenterologist who did not take a history took a colon biopsy specimen that showed mucosal edema, congestion, and numerous lymphoid cells in the lamina propria. Which of the following differential diagnoses would apply?

(A) Staphylococcal gastroenteritis vs. Crohn's disease
(B) Viral gastroenteritis vs. acute diverticulitis
(C) Colonic endometriosis vs. amebic dysentery
(D) Early ulcerative colitis vs. *Salmonella* colitis
(E) Bleeding hemorrhoids vs. Meckel's diverticulitis

251. A 32-year-old woman sees her physician because of "stiffness" and intolerance to cold temperatures in her fingers. Her face has a "mask-like" quality. It would be appropriate in the systems review to ask about

(A) headaches and dizziness
(B) swallowing difficulties
(C) sun hypersensitivity
(D) thyroid trouble
(E) family history

252. The lesion seen in the photomicrograph below is referred to as

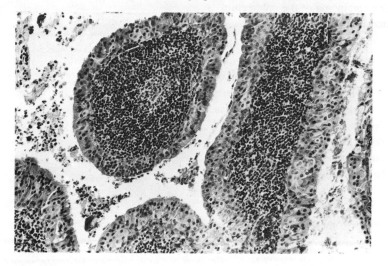

(A) adenoid cystic carcinoma
(B) lymphoepithelioma
(C) thyroglossal duct neoplasm
(D) Warthin's tumor
(E) sebaceous lymphadenoma

---

253. All the following statements concerning carcinoma of the stomach are true EXCEPT

(A) there is a striking geographical variation in death rate from gastric carcinoma
(B) *early gastric carcinoma (EGC)* is synonymous with *carcinoma in situ*
(C) over 50 percent of gastric carcinomas are found in the pylorus and antrum
(D) diffusely infiltrative carcinoma is associated with a striking desmoplastic reaction
(E) the death rate from gastric carcinoma has been decreasing for decades

254. All the following statements regarding carcinoma of the esophagus are true EXCEPT

(A) most carcinomas arising in the body of the esophagus are squamous
(B) squamous carcinomas begin as lesions in situ
(C) patients with Barrett's esophagus have approximately a 10 percent risk of carcinoma
(D) the most common morphologic form is a polypoid fungating mass
(E) distant metastases are frequently present at the time of diagnosis

255. All the following statements concerning carcinoma of the colorectum
are true EXCEPT

(A) 95 percent of all carcinomas of the
     colorectum are adenocarcinoma
(B) mucin secretion aids extension of
     the primary malignancy
(C) left-sided lesions tend to grow as
     polypoid fungating masses
(D) serum levels of carcinoembryonic
     antigen (CEA) are directly related
     to size and spread
(E) serum levels of CEA fall to zero
     with complete removal of the
     tumor

256. The photomicrograph below was prepared after a distal colonic biopsy was
performed. The most likely diagnosis is

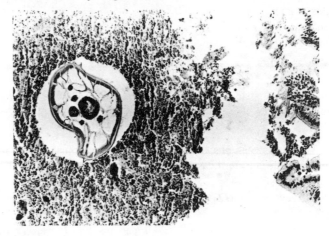

(A) clonorchiasis
(B) enterobiasis
(C) filariasis
(D) strongyloidiasis
(E) schistosomiasis

257. In the photograph below, an ulcerated mucosal lesion is shown at the anorectal junction. This lesion is

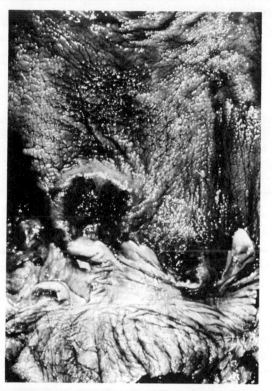

(A) a villous adenoma
(B) a basaloid carcinoma
(C) a hemorrhoid
(D) a polypoid adenoma
(E) a mesenteric thrombus

258. A mononuclear portal inflammatory infiltrate that disrupts the limiting plate and surrounds individual hepatocytes (piecemeal necrosis), as shown in the photomicrograph below, is characteristic of

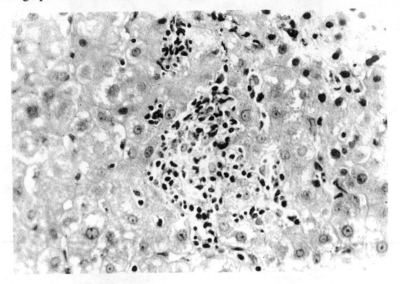

(A) ascending cholangitis
(B) chronic active hepatitis
(C) acute alcoholic hepatitis
(D) cholestatic jaundice
(E) nutritional cirrhosis

259. A middle-aged patient is undergoing surgical exploration for a tumor in the pancreatic fundus. No clinical history is given to the pathologist, who notes that the tumor has an "endocrine" appearance in frozen section. An appropriate step in the subsequent evaluation would be to consider

(A) immunoperoxidase
(B) brain scans
(C) computerized tomography
(D) celiac angiography
(E) immunofluorescence testing

260. A middle-aged male alcoholic has had repeated bouts of pancreatitis following periods of binge drinking. In recent months he has had a low-grade fever, and on examination a mass is palpated in the epigastrium. This mass, removed at celiotomy, is shown in the photograph below. What is the diagnosis?

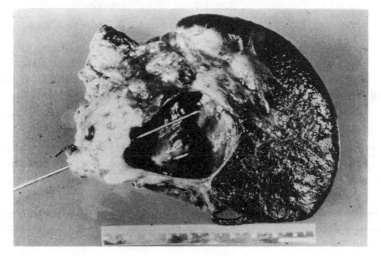

(A) Pancreatic carcinoma
(B) Mucinous cystadenoma
(C) Perforated ulcer
(D) Pancreatic pseudocyst
(E) Cystic hepatoma

261. Two subtotal colectomy specimens are sent to the laboratory with both showing a hemorrhagic cobblestone appearance of the mucosa. One, however, shows longitudinal grooving of the surface, which suggests

(A) ischemic bowel disease
(B) multiple polyposis syndrome
(C) ulcerative colitis
(D) Crohn's disease
(E) none of the above

DIRECTIONS: Each question below contains four suggested responses of which **one or more** is correct. Select

A	if	**1, 2, and 3**	are correct
B	if	**1 and 3**	are correct
C	if	**2 and 4**	are correct
D	if	**4**	is correct
E	if	**1, 2, 3, and 4**	are correct

262. True statements regarding congenital pyloric stenosis include that it

(1) occurs predominantly in male infants
(2) is manifested during the first few days of life
(3) is manifested by vomiting, dehydration, and malnutrition
(4) resolves spontaneously, but symptomatic medical management should be promptly instituted

263. Carcinoma of the exocrine pancreas

(1) is predominantly adenocarcinoma
(2) is more common in diabetics than in nondiabetics
(3) may be associated with fluctuating levels of jaundice
(4) is usually not widely disseminated at autopsy

264. True statements regarding peptic ulceration include that

(1) hyperparathyroidism is a predisposing factor
(2) in Zollinger-Ellison syndrome up to 25 percent of ulcers are in atypical location
(3) mucosa adjacent to ulcers frequently shows intestinal metaplasia
(4) the base of a peptic ulcer contains necrotic debris

265. Tumors of the salivary glands are characterized by which of the following statements?

(1) They are principally epithelial in origin
(2) When malignant, they tend to metastasize early and pursue a rapid course
(3) They tend to present similarly, regardless of histological pattern
(4) They are less likely to be malignant in the minor salivary glands than in the parotids

266. The photomicrograph below shows a section through the wall of the gall-bladder. True statements regarding the condition illustrated include that

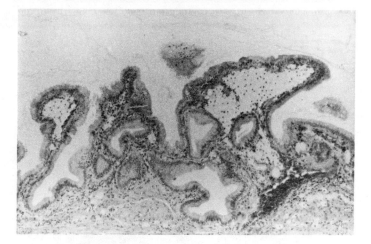

(1) it is commonly associated with gallstones
(2) it is associated with mural calcification
(3) it may mimic a tumor of the gallbladder radiologically
(4) it predisposes to acute cholecystitis

---

267. Angiodysplasia of the colon is known to be an important cause of unexplained anemia or lower gastrointestinal bleeding in the elderly. It is associated with

(1) occurrence in the descending colon
(2) dilated mucosal and submucosal veins
(3) portal hypertension
(4) diagnosis by colonoscopy and angiography

SUMMARY OF DIRECTIONS

A	B	C	D	E
1, 2, 3 only	1, 3 only	2, 4 only	4 only	All are correct

268.   Which of the following statements would correctly characterize the colonic lesion shown in the photograph below?

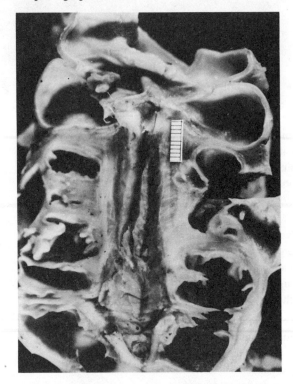

(1)   The prevalence is highest in people under 50 years of age
(2)   The lesions are more common in women than in men
(3)   Colonic lesions occur most frequently in the ascending and transverse segments of the colon
(4)   The lesions occur more commonly in the colon than in other portions of the gastrointestinal tract

269. True statements regarding alcoholic steatosis and hepatitis as illustrated in the photomicrograph below include

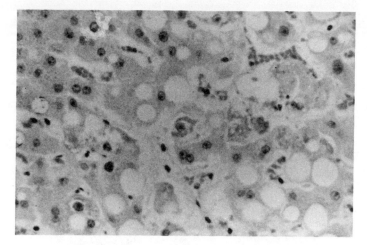

(1) morphological changes of steatosis are irreversible
(2) changes in hepatitis are most marked around portal tracts
(3) Mallory's hyaline is pathognomonic of alcoholic liver damage
(4) perivenular and pericellular fibroses are precursors of cirrhosis

---

270. A 65-year-old man presents with episodes of facial flushing exacerbated by alcohol and associated with severe diarrhea. Which of the following findings would be expected on evaluation and treatment of this patient?

(1) Increased urinary levels of 5-hydroxyindoleacetic acid (5-HIAA)
(2) Elevated levels of serotonin in circulating platelets
(3) Areas of decreased uptake on liver scintillation scan
(4) A small yellow nodule in the tip of the appendix, found at laparotomy

271. Anemia may be associated with gastric malignancies as the result of

(1) tumor ulceration of vascular structures
(2) achlorhydria with decreased intrinsic factor
(3) marrow myelophthisis secondary to bone marrow metastases
(4) iron malabsorption

SUMMARY OF DIRECTIONS

A	B	C	D	E
1, 2, 3 only	1, 3 only	2, 4 only	4 only	All are correct

272. Finely nodular (micronodular) cirrhosis, as evident in the photomicrograph below, is usually associated with

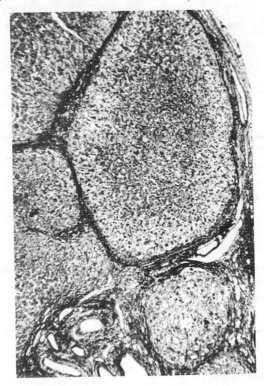

(1) massive hepatic necrosis
(2) increased fat within hepatocytes
(3) viral hepatitis
(4) alcohol abuse

273. Cell types that are found, alone or in combination, in gastric carcinoma include

(1) epithelial mucous cells
(2) parietal cells
(3) metaplastic intestinal cells
(4) enterochromaffin cells

274. In primary biliary cirrhosis, abnormal results are found in which of the following?

(1) Serum IgM
(2) Alkaline phosphatase
(3) Serum copper level
(4) Mitochondrial antibody test

---

275. The gross photograph below shows a portion of a liver removed during emergency surgery from a 26-year-old woman who had abdominal pain and an acute (surgical) abdomen on examination and who had been taking birth control pills. This disorder

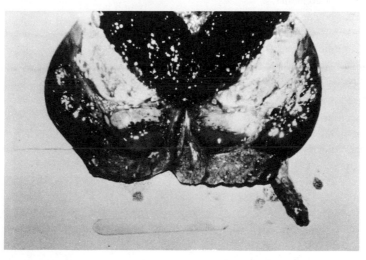

(1) also occurs in infants and men
(2) was rare before birth control pills were introduced
(3) shows an absence of bile ducts
(4) includes hematoma formation

SUMMARY OF DIRECTIONS

A	B	C	D	E
1, 2, 3 only	1, 3 only	2, 4 only	4 only	All are correct

276. In a needle biopsy of the liver, diseases likely to be confused with cirrhosis include

(1) mesenchymal hamartoma
(2) infantile hemangioendothelioma
(3) liver cell adenoma
(4) focal nodular hyperplasia

277. Conditions that may produce ulceroinflammatory changes confined to the anorectal area include

(1) Crohn's disease
(2) infection with *Treponema pallidum*
(3) idiopathic ulcerative proctitis
(4) tuberculosis

278. Pancreatitis is commonly associated with which of the following?

(1) Stones in the ampulla of Vater
(2) A history of alcoholism
(3) Cholecystitis
(4) Hypertension

279. Whipple's disease (intestinal lipodystrophy) is an uncommon disorder that is associated with

(1) steatorrhea
(2) emaciation
(3) enlarged mucosal and mesenteric lymph nodes
(4) atrophic intestinal mucosa

DIRECTIONS: Each group of questions below consists of four lettered headings followed by a set of numbered items. For each numbered item select

A	if the item is associated with	(A) **only**
B	if the item is associated with	(B) **only**
C	if the item is associated with	**both** (A) and (B)
D	if the item is associated with	**neither** (A) nor (B)

Each lettered heading may be used **once, more than once, or not at all.**

Questions 280-282

(A) Ulcerative colitis
(B) Crohn's disease
(C) Both
(D) Neither

280. Erythema nodosum

281. Crypt abscesses

282. Fibrinomucinous exudate

Questions 283-286

(A) Primary biliary cirrhosis
(B) Laennec's cirrhosis
(C) Both
(D) Neither

283. Alcohol abuse

284. Bile duct proliferation

285. Xanthomas of skin and ulcerative colitis

286. Equal sex incidence

DIRECTIONS: The group of questions below consists of lettered headings followed by a set of numbered items. For each numbered item select the **one** lettered heading with which it is **most** closely associated. Each lettered heading may be used **once, more than once, or not at all.**

Questions 287-290

Match each of the clinical and pathological patterns of malabsorption syndrome with the appropriate cause.

(A) Abetalipoproteinemia
(B) Primary intestinal lymphoma
(C) Whipple's disease
(D) Disaccharidase deficiency
(E) Systemic mastocytosis

287. Recent viral infection, persistent diarrhea, normal bowel mucosa

288. Arthralgias, lymphadenopathy, blunted villi distended by macrophages

289. Diarrhea unresponsive to gluten-free diet, blunted villi with chronic inflammatory infiltrate

290. Failure to thrive, steatorrhea, lipid vacuolation of mucosal cells

Gastrointestinal System
Answers

249. The answer is D. *(Rosai, ed 7. pp 577-580.)* The condition illustrated is ulcerative colitis, an inflammatory disorder of unknown cause. It involves the distal colon with variable proximal extension. Grossly there is ulceration with islands of residual mucosa. The inflammation is predominantly superficial with an infiltrate of acute and chronic inflammatory cells in the lamina propria. Cryptitis and crypt abscesses are common. Many lymphoid follicles may be seen but epithelioid cells, giant cells, and granulomas are absent. Cellular atypia is seen in regenerating mucosa. Submucosal arteries show features of endarteritis obliterans in approximately 10 percent of cases. When ulcerative colitis is inactive, morphologic abnormalities of glands, goblet cell depletion, and Paneth cell metaplasia indicate underlying disease.

250. The answer is D. *(Robbins, ed 4. pp 353-355, 867-869, 886-889.)* Early stages of ulcerative colitis (UC) may be indistinguishable from gastroenteritis caused by *Salmonella choleraesuis* and *S. typhimurium*. In early stages, both diseases may show histologically a dense mononuclear inflammatory infiltrate in the lamina propria, occasional crypt abscesses, and mucosal edema and congestion. Even the respective clinical symptoms and colon x-ray changes may be similar, although marked vomiting should point to food poisoning. Salmonellae have been the cause of outbreaks and epidemics of acute gastroenteritis, and the cause has often been found to be contaminated fowl that has been insufficiently cooked to inactivate endotoxins.

251. The answer is B. *(Robbins ed 4. pp 204-207, 579.)* The constellation of Raynaud's phenomenon, acral sclerosis, and fibrotic tightening of the muscles of facial expression should raise the specter of progressive systemic sclerosis (scleroderma), a multisystem disease that involves the cardiovascular, gastrointestinal, cutaneous, musculoskeletal, pulmonary, and renal systems through progressive interstitial fibrosis. Small arterioles in the forenamed systems show obliteration caused by intimal hyperplasia accompanied by progressive interstitial fibrosis. Evidence implicates a lymphocyte overdrive of fibroblasts to produce an excess of rather normal collagen. Eventually, myocardial fibrosis, pulmonary fibrosis, and terminal renal failure ensue. Over half of all patients have dysphagia with solid food caused by the distal esophageal narrowing in the disease.

252. The answer is D. *(Robbins, ed 4. pp 824-826.)* Warthin's tumors occur mainly in the lower regions of the parotid gland, especially near the angle of the mandible, and on rare occasion may be bilateral. They are completely benign neoplasms although they carry some undesirable synonyms: *adenolymphoma*, which is a misnomer, and *papillary cystadenoma lymphomatosum*, a term undesirable both for the *lymphomatosum* part as well as its length. For these reasons most workers prefer the term *Warthin's tumor*. The pattern is highly characteristic of an epithelial surface lining of acidophilic cells that overlay benign lymphoid tissue elements, including germinal centers. The epithelial portion probably arises from early duct cells that become entrapped within developing parotid lymph nodes during embryogenesis. Sebaceous lymphadenoma would have sebaceous cells within the lymphoid tissue. Thyroglossal duct cyst is located in the midline of the neck but may be found extending up to the base of the tongue, and there is a similarity between the lymphoid islands seen in thyroglossal duct cysts and in Warthin's tumor; however, thyroid follicles may lead to the correct diagnosis in the former. Lymphoepithelioma is a tumor that is recognized by hyperplastic duct epithelium surrounded by lymphoid tissue. Myoepithelial islands embedded in lymphoid tissue may be seen in the minor and major salivary glands in Sjögren's syndrome.

253. The answer is B. *(Robbins, ed 4. pp 854-858.)* The death rate from gastric carcinoma has been decreasing for decades, but still shows marked variations among countries; Japan, Chile, and Iceland have rates up to six times higher than that of the U.S. and Australia. First-generation migrants carry the risk of their country of origin, but subsequent generations assume the risk of their new country. *Early gastric carcinoma (EGC)* refers to a local neoplastic lesion limited to the mucosa and submucosa without penetration of the muscularis propria. Metastasis can occur, however, from EGC to local lymph nodes in up to 5 percent of cases. EGC is usually recognizable on radiographic or endoscopic examination, and so in most cases is potentially curable. It develops very slowly into a frankly invasive lesion and, if detected early and removed, allows a 5-year survival of up to 95 percent compared with 15 percent for gastric carcinoma overall. Of all gastric carcinomas, 50 to 60 percent arise in the pyloro-antrum, 10 percent in the cardia, 10 percent in the whole organ, and the remainder in other sites. Diffusely infiltrating carcinoma extends widely through the stomach wall, often without producing an intraluminal mass, and incites a marked desmoplastic reaction that results in a thickened, inelastic stomach wall.

254. The answer is E. *(Robbins, ed 4. pp 835-838.)* Carcinoma of the esophagus accounts for about 10 percent of malignancies of the GI tract, but for a disproportionate number of cancer deaths. Predisposing factors include smoking, esophagitis, and achalasia. Sixty to seventy percent are squamous cell carcinomas that characteristically begin as lesions in situ. Adenocarcinoma occurs mainly in the lower esophagus and may arise in up to 10 percent of cases of Barrett's esophagus. Anaplastic and small-cell variants also occur. Polypoid lesions are most common, followed by malignant ulceration and diffusively infiltrative forms. Tumors tend to spread by direct invasion of adjacent structures, but lymphatic and hematogenous spread may occur. Distant metastases are, however, a late feature. Five-year survival is less than 10 percent.

255. The answer is C. *(Robbins, ed 4. pp 897-901.)* Ninety-five percent of all carcinomas of the colorectum are adenocarcinoma. The remainder are adenosquamous or adenoacanthoma. Many of the adenocarcinomas secrete mucin. When this secretion is extracellular, it dissects the gut wall cell planes and so aids extension of the malignancy. The gross pathology of left- and right-sided lesions differs; left-sided lesions tend to grow in an annular encircling fashion, while right-sided lesions tend to be sessile or polypoid fungating masses. Carcinoembryonic antigen is the tumor marker longest used in diagnosis and follow-up of colorectal tumors. Its serum levels are directly related to both size and extent of spread of the primary tumor. With large neoplasms there is almost 100 percent positivity. Levels fall to zero with complete removal of tumor but rise again with recurrence at primary or secondary sites.

256. The answer is B. *(Anderson, ed 9. pp 161 165.)* In the photomicrograph, a cross section of an *Enterobius* adult worm is shown. Apparent morphologic features of this nematode include the bilateral crests, the meromyarial type of musculature, and the noncellular cuticle with spines. *Enterobius vermicularis,* the agent responsible for the helminthic infection most common in the United States, usually produces pruritus ani as the outstanding and most disturbing symptom of enterobiasis (pinworm infection). *Enterobius* worms often attach themselves to the cecal mucosa and contiguous regions, but the usual host sites for schistosomiasis, clonorchiasis, and filariasis are the veins of the large intestine, the bile ducts, and the lymphatics, respectively. Elephantiasis is a characteristic feature in filariasis, and infection by *Strongyloides stercoralis* usually produces hyperemia and edema of the small intestinal mucosa.

257. The answer is B. *(Robbins, ed 4. p 902.)* The lesion pictured is a basaloid or cloacogenic carcinoma that has the same gross appearance as the more common epidermoid carcinoma, although the lesion histologically resembles the basal cell carcinoma of the skin. The tumor arises from the anal canal within the transitional zone epithelium (anal columns). Some of these tumors resemble transitional epithelium, whereas others vary in their patterns, including one pattern similar to that of small-cell (oat cell) carcinoma of the lung and other patterns that are totally undifferentiated. The prognosis for cloacogenic carcinoma is directly proportional to the degree of differentiation.

258. The answer is B. *(Robbins, ed 4. pp 924-937.)* Chronic hepatitis has been defined as an inflammatory process of the liver that lasts longer than 1 year and lacks the nodular regeneration and architectural distortion of cirrhosis. In chronic active hepatitis, an intense inflammatory reaction with numerous plasma cells spreads from portal tracts into periportal areas. The reaction destroys the limiting plate and results in formation of periportal hepatocytic islets. Prognosis is poor, and the majority of patients develop cirrhosis. Chronic persistent hepatitis is usually a sequela of acute viral hepatitis and has a benign course, without progression to chronic active hepatitis or cirrhosis. The portal inflammation does not extend into the periportal areas, thus differentiating it from chronic active hepatitis.

259. The answer is A. *(Robbins, ed 4. pp 1005-1008. Schwarz, N Engl J Med 305:917, 1981.)* Any tumor of the pancreas seen to have an organoid (endocrine-like) pattern histologically, even in frozen section, should arouse suspicion of an islet cell tumor, a carcinoid, or a component tumor of multiple endocrine neoplasia. The pathologist may be alert to this possibility if appropriate clinical information relating the patient's symptoms accompanies the biopsy specimen. Electron microscopy will show specialized types of electron-dense core granules ("neurosecretory" granules) in the cytoplasm in the presence of tumors of the amine precursor uptake decarboxylation class (APUDomas). Islet cell tumors may contain alpha (glucagon), beta (insulin), delta (somatostatin), and pp (pancreatic polypeptide) dense-core granules. Direct staining of the hormones can be accomplished with immunoperoxidase, which contains the specific antibody to the hormone being sought and forms rust-brown granules that can be seen with the ordinary light microscope.

260. The answer is D. *(Robbins, ed 4. pp 988-989.)* Pseudocysts of the pancreas are so named because the cystic structure is essentially unlined by any type of epithelium. True cysts, wherever they are found in the body, are always lined by some type of epithelium, whether columnar cell, glandular, squamous, or flattened cuboidal cell. The pancreatic pseudocyst is most commonly found in a background of repeated episodes of pancreatitis. Eventual mechanical large duct obstruction by either an inflammatory process per se, periductal fibrosis, or an abscess along with inspissated duct fluid from secretions and enzymes leads to the expanding mass. The mass lesion may be located between the stomach and liver, between the stomach and colon or transverse mesocolon, or in the lesser sac. Drainage or excision is necessary for adequate treatment. Acute bacterial infection may complicate the course.

261. The answer is D. *(Robbins, ed 4. pp 868-872.)* Hemorrhagic cobblestone appearance of the colon and small bowel may be seen in multiple states including inflammatory bowel disease, a term that can apply both to ulcerative colitis and regional enteritis (Crohn's disease). Other conditions that resemble cobblestoning of the mucosa of the bowel include multiple polyps such as occur in Gardner's syndrome, Turcot syndrome, familial polyposis, and multiple acquired polyps. Crohn's disease, however, differs from the others in that longitudinal ulcers may be present, yielding a long axis grooving, parallel to the long axis of the bowel. Such ulcers may also be seen in tuberculous enteritis; however, when inflammatory bowel disease is in the differential diagnosis, longitudinal ulcers are indicative of Crohn's disease.

262. The answer is B (1, 3). *(Robbins, ed 4. pp 841-842.)* Congenital pyloric stenosis is seen predominantly in male infants at the age of approximately 3 weeks. The pyloric lumen is narrowed by pronounced smooth muscle hypertrophy. Vomiting is seen following feedings and is remarkably projectile in view of the infant's age. In some cases, the pyloric area is palpable on abdominal examination. There is a classic "double-bubble" radiologic sign. The only cure is surgery.

263. The answer is E (all). *(Robbins, ed 4. pp 990-992.)* Carcinoma of the exocrine pancreas has a higher rate of incidence in males, blacks, smokers, chemists exposed to beta naphthylamine, and diabetics. It is predominantly adenocarcinoma, although 10 percent are adenosquamous or anaplastic tumors, and 0.5 percent are cystadenocarcinomas. Although it invades ducts, destroys islets, and invades vessels and lymphatics, it causes death from hepatobiliary dysfunction at an early stage and so is usually not widely disseminated at autopsy. It is often thought to be associated with progressive and unremitting jaundice, but areas of necrosis within the tumor may allow transient bile flow and hence fluctuating levels of jaundice.

264. The answer is A (1, 2, 3). *(Robbins, ed 4. pp 845-853, 1007.)* Peptic ulceration can occur in any area of the gastrointestinal tract exposed to acid-pepsin. In Zollinger-Ellison syndrome it occurs in the stomach and in atypical locations in the duodenum and jejunum. Predisposing factors include cirrhosis, chronic renal failure, chronic obstructive pulmonary disease (COPD), hyperparathyroidism, hypercalcemia, and therapy with nonsteroidal anti-inflammatory drugs (NSAIDs). *Campylobacter pyloris* breaks down glycoproteins in the gastric mucus, which favors development of chronic gastritis and possible gastric ulcers. Peptic ulcers are sharply punched-out defects of varying depth with a smooth and clean base due to peptic digestion of exudate. The surrounding mucosa is edematous and shows regeneration, frequently with intestinal metaplasia.

265. The answer is B (1, 3). *(Robbins, ed 4. pp 822-826.)* The salivary glands give rise to a wide variety of tumors. The majority are benign, chiefly pleomorphic adenomas. From 75 to 85 percent occur in the parotids, 10 to 20 percent in the submandibulars, and the remainder in the minor glands. In the parotids up to 80 percent are benign, whereas in the palatal glands benign and malignant tumors occur with equal frequency. It is evident, therefore, that a tumor is more likely to be malignant in the minor glands than in the parotid. Up to 95 percent of tumors of the salivary glands are epithelial in origin, although some have lymphoid components. Mesenchymal malignancies are rare. Clinically, tumors of the salivary glands tend to present similarly regardless of histological pattern. Most present as palpable masses, usually in the parotid. They may occasionally present with symptoms related to local invasion, such as facial nerve palsies. Masses may be present for years before diagnosis, even when malignant. Diagnosis often depends on excision and analysis. Carcinomas tend to run a slow course, invading local structures slowly, recurring locally after removal, and metastasizing late. Prognosis is usually quoted in 10- or 20-year survival rates.

266. The answer is B (1, 3). *(Robbins, ed 4. p 973.)* The condition shown is cholesterolosis, also known as "strawberry gallbladder" (owing to its gross appearance). It is a fairly common condition, but is of little clinical significance and is not thought to predispose to acute cholecystitis, although it is commonly associated with cholesterol calculi. Cholesterol is taken up by mucosal histiocytes, which become distended and have foamy cytoplasm. They distend the mucosal folds of the gallbladder and, in extreme cases, can lead to a polypoid mass, which may mimic a tumor on cholecystography. Mural calcification (porcelain gallbladder) may develop in chronic cholecystitis but shows no association with cholesterolosis. There is an increased risk of gallbladder cancer with mural calcification.

267. The answer is C (2, 4). *(Robbins, ed 4. pp 885-886.)* Angiodysplasia of the colon is characterized by dilated, tortuous, submucosal veins and mucosal venules in the cecum and ascending colon. These venous abnormalities apparently result from long-term tension of the cecal wall that causes intermittent occlusion of the thin-walled veins and thus raises pressures in these submucosal and mucosal veins with eventual dilatation and possible rupture. Angiodysplasia does not occur in other parts of the colon. Such mucosal vascular dilatation can only be diagnosed by colonoscopy, which shows mucosal vascular "blushes," and selective mesenteric angiography. Portal hypertension is occasionally associated with development of hemorrhoids as collateral anastomotic channels with protrusion of varices beneath anal or rectal mucosa.

268. The answer is D (4). *(Anderson, ed 9. p 1155.)* Diverticula occur most frequently in men over the age of 50 in the descending and sigmoid colon. The colon is the most commonly involved segment of the gastrointestinal tract. A majority of these lesions are not "true" diverticula, since the mucosa and muscularis mucosa herniate through defects in the muscular wall.

269. The answer is D (4). *(Robbins, ed 4. pp 944-949. Rosai, ed 7. pp 684-687.)* Alcoholic liver disease includes alcoholic steatosis (fatty liver), alcoholic hepatitis, and cirrhosis. Steatosis is the earliest hepatic consequence of excess alcohol intake and consists of cytoplasmic accumulation of lipid vacuoles, which coalesce to distend hepatocytes with ultrastructural evidence of cell injury. However, these changes are completely reversible. Alcoholic hepatitis is usually accompanied by some fatty change and is characterized by hepatocellular swelling, necrosis, and neutrophil infiltration in the centrilobular area, as well as the appearance of Mallory's hyaline—

eosinophilic cytoplasmic inclusions composed of keratin proteins. These inclusions are characteristic of alcoholic injury, but may occur in primary biliary cirrhosis, biliary obstruction, and other diseases. Pericellular fibrosis and fibrosis around the central vein are significant changes considered by some to indicate the possible development of cirrhosis.

270. The answer is A (1, 2, 3). *(Robbins, ed 4. pp 872-875.)* The patient shows two of the most common clinical manifestations of the carcinoid syndrome. Flushing is found in 90 percent, diarrhea in 75 percent, bronchoconstriction in 20 percent, and right-sided endocardial fibrosis in 35 percent of patients with the carcinoid syndrome. Carcinoid syndrome results from elaboration of serotonin by a primary carcinoid tumor in the lung or ovary, or liver metastases from a gastrointestinal carcinoid. Diagnosis is based on finding increased urinary 5-HIAA from metabolism of excess serotonin, and on histological analysis of tumor tissue found at laparotomy. Primary appendiceal carcinoid metastasizes in approximately 0.2 percent of cases and is virtually always asymptomatic.

271. The answer is A (1, 2, 3). *(Robbins, ed 4. pp 843-845.)* Atrophic gastritis is commonly associated with gastric carcinoma and regularly occurs concomitantly with pernicious anemia. Decreased HCl secretion (or achlorhydria) results from the decrease in number or absence of parietal cells that is typical in gastric atrophy. Pernicious anemia is also associated with achlorhydria. Blood loss from ulcerating tumor masses is common throughout the gastrointestinal tract. Since most iron is absorbed in the small intestine, iron malabsorption would not be directly associated with gastric tumors.

272. The answer is C (2, 4). *(Robbins, ed 4. pp 944-949.)* Chronic alcohol abuse may lead to Laennec's (micronodular) cirrhosis and is usually accompanied by fat accumulation. In massive hepatic necrosis from viral hepatitis or drug or chemical toxicity, the pattern of scarring and regeneration is random, scars are broad, and nodules form that are 3 to 4 cm in diameter. In alcoholic cirrhosis the lobules are regenerated liver parenchyma lacking central veins (pseudolobules).

273. The answer is B (1, 3). *(Robbins, ed 4. pp 856-857.)* Gastric carcinomas are all composed of two basic cell types: gastric mucous cells and intestinal metaplastic cells. Mucous cells are tall columnar cells that form the surface lining of the stomach. They secrete a mucopolysaccharide mucin. Both cell types may show mucin vacuoles, which may distort cellular architecture and produce "signet-ring cells." Mucin may also surround cells or glands and aid local spread of tumor. Metaplastic intestinal cells contain mucin that may be gastric or intestinal in character. They contain enzymes not found in normal gastric epithelium, such as alkaline phosphatase and beta glucuronidase. Parietal cells are found in the neck and isthmic regions of gastric glands. They secrete hydrochloric acid. Enterochromaffin cells are small cells with

APUD characteristics. They are involved in the production and release of polypeptides and protein hormones. If malignant, they are found in carcinoid tumors.

274. The answer is E (all). *(Anderson, ed 9. pp 1255-1257.)* In the United States and in Europe primary biliary cirrhosis predominantly involves middle-aged women (a mean age of 52). It is characterized clinically by an insidious clinical course starting with pruritus, which gives way eventually to jaundice and hyperlipemia manifested by xanthomas of the palms of the hands, the arms, and the eyelids. The laboratory findings include a positive antimitochondrial antibody, elevated IgM, elevated alkaline phosphatase, hyperglobulinemia, elevated serum copper levels, and circulating immune complexes. Sjögren's syndrome is increased in this disorder as are some of the other collagen vascular diseases, including scleroderma, lupus erythematosus, and thyroiditis. Histopathologic changes of the liver include portal triaditis with destruction of the limiting plate and of the bile ducts with eventual replacement of the portal triads by cirrhosis and a loss of bile ducts. Granulomas and xanthomatous giant cells are frequently seen.

275. The answer is E (all). *(Anderson, ed 9. pp 1289-1290.)* Hepatic adenomas (HAs) did occur before the introduction of oral contraceptive pills in the 1960s. Furthermore, these adenomas of liver cells do occur in women not taking birth control pills, infants, children, and even men, but they are exceedingly rare in these patients, and accompanying hemorrhage with hematoma formation appears not to occur unless the patient has been using birth control pills. Women taking oral contraceptives (mestranol) who develop liver cell adenomas are at risk of hemorrhage with rupture into the abdominal cavity and exsanguination. Microscopically, bile duct branches are not present in HAs, which helps to distinguish them from focal nodular hyperplasia of the liver, which is seen primarily in adult women.

276. The answer is D (4). *(Robbins, ed 4. pp 957-958.)* Focal nodular hyperplasia is likely to be confused with nutritional or alcoholic cirrhosis and on occasion, depending on the stage, with primary biliary cirrhosis. Focal nodular hyperplasia is most likely a hamartoma and is recognized by a stellate scar formation grossly, which microscopically demonstrates increased fibrous connective tissue with scattered bile ductules and regenerative nodules of liver cells. Liver cell adenoma does not contain an increase in bile ducts and most often they are even absent. Hemangioendotheliomas in the liver in childhood show fibrosis and an increase in bile ducts, which are found at the periphery mainly with small capillaries throughout the lesion mixed with prominent endothelial cells. The mesenchymal hamartoma of the liver also has a fibrous stromal bed but has alternating clusters of proliferative bile ducts with epithelial cells distributed in an island-like fashion throughout the lesion. There have been questions raised concerning the relationship of focal nodular hyperplasia to oral contraceptives, but the evidence is less than clear. Of interest is the fact that Felty's syndrome has been reported in association with focal nodular hyperplasia.

277. The answer is A (1, 2, 3). *(Braunwald, ed 11. pp 516, 1280-1282. Robbins, ed 4. pp 866-867.)* Ulceroinflammatory changes in the colon occur in a variety of conditions. In some they may be limited to the anorectal area. Crohn's disease may induce proctitis without affecting more proximal areas of the gut. Infectious agents such as *Treponema pallidum,* gonococcus, chlamydia, and herpes simplex cause an isolated proctitis that is found particularly in male homosexuals. Idiopathic ulcerative proctitis is a nonspecific rectal mucosal inflammation that causes painless rectal bleeding, diarrhea, and tenesmus. The rectal mucosa is friable, granular, and ulcerated on proctoscopy. Microscopic appearance is similar to that of ulcerative colitis, and some authorities hold that it is the benign end of the spectrum of ulcerative colitis. With inflammation confined to the rectum, risk of developing carcinoma is negligible. Tuberculosis typically produces transverse ulcers with overhanging margins in the ileocecal region.

278. The answer is A (1, 2, 3). *(Anderson, ed 9. pp 1351-1353.)* Most of the postulated etiologic factors for pancreatitis invoke mechanisms of partial or complete obstruction of the pancreatic duct and increased pancreatic secretion. Malignant hypertension may cause vascular necroses in the pancreas, but only focal necrosis of pancreatic tissue occurs, not general pancreatitis.

279. The answer is A (1, 2, 3). *(Anderson, ed 9. pp 1173-1174.)* Whipple's disease (intestinal lipodystrophy) is characterized by steatorrhea, accumulation of lipids in lacteals and in mucosal and mesenteric lymph nodes, and deposition of PAS-positive carbohydrate-protein complexes in histiocytes within the lamina propria of the intestinal villi and in other tissues. Although the villi of the small intestine become blunted and distended by masses of histiocytes, the mucosa is not atrophic. Patients who have Whipple's disease are emaciated and often have gray-brown melanin pigmentation of the skin. Evaluation of an intestinal biopsy to detect glycoprotein-laden histiocytes in the villi may be necessary to confirm a diagnosis because patients often have many nonspecific systemic symptoms.

280-282. The answers are: 280-C, 281-A, 282-D. *(Robbins, ed 4. pp 869-871, 887-889.)* Ulcerative colitis and Crohn's disease may show very similar morphological features. Useful findings in distinguishing the two include total colonic involvement, distal predominance, broad-based ulcers, pseudopolyps, and crypt abscesses, all of which are more frequently found in ulcerative colitis; and skip lesions, serpentine fissures, transmural inflammation, lymphoid aggregates, granulomas, and fibrous thickening, which suggest a diagnosis of Crohn's disease. Extragastrointestinal manifestations such as erythema nodosum, arthritis, uveitis, pericholangitis, and ankylosing spondylitis may be associated with both ulcerative colitis and Crohn's disease. Fissures and cutaneous fistulas in the perineum are suggestive of Crohn's disease, rather than ulcerative colitis. A fibrinomucinous exudate that appears to erupt from the mucosal crypts and is associated with a normal or hyperemic mucosa is found in pseudomembranous colitis (PMC). PMC is usually caused by the toxin of *Clostridium difficile,* although it may also result from infection by staphylococcus, shigella, or candida, or from ischemia. Most often it occurs after broad-spectrum antibiotics—such as clindamycin, lincomycin, or ampicillin—have been given.

283-286. The answers are: 283-B, 284-C, 285-A, 286-D. *(Anderson, ed 9. pp 1208-1210, 1244-1247, 1254-1257.)* Alcohol abuse, alcoholic hepatitis, and Laennec's (micronodular) cirrhosis are closely related. Cirrhosis of alcoholic liver disease is characterized by micronodules of regenerated hepatocytes surrounded by peripheral fibrosis. Central veins are only rarely seen within the pseudonodules. The fibrotic network contains varying bile duct proliferation and chronic inflammatory cells.

Atypical bile duct proliferation is a diagnostic feature of primary biliary cirrhosis (PBC), although it also occurs in Laennec's cirrhosis. High levels of serum cholesterol result in dermal xanthomas and ulcerative colitis and are associated with PBC. PBC presents in middle-aged women, who experience pruritus, jaundice, and nontender hepatomegaly. Alkaline phosphatase levels in the serum are elevated, and antimitochondrial antibodies can be demonstrated. There is evidence that PBC is autoimmune, with sensitized T cells involved in the granulomatous and bile duct inflammatory lesions. There is a gradual loss of intrahepatic bile ducts after an initial stage of lymphocytic and granulomatous inflammation. This is followed by a stage of bile duct proliferation. The third stage is active fibrosis.

Laennec's cirrhosis occurs more frequently in men. Primary biliary cirrhosis occurs much more frequently in women (9:1 ratio).

287-290. The answers are: 287-D, 288-C, 289-B, 290-A. *(Braunwald, ed 11. pp 1264-1272. Robbins, ed 4. pp 875-881.)* Malabsorption syndromes have protean causes and are broadly categorized on the basis of the underlying abnormality. Abetalipoproteinemia is a rare condition in which absence of lipoprotein-B leads to inability to synthesize prebetalipoproteins (VLDL), betalipoproteins (LDL), and chylomicrons. Consequently, lipid accumulates in vacuoles in mucosal cells.

Whipple's disease is a multisystem disorder of presumed infectious origin. The lamina propria of the small intestinal mucosa is distended by PAS-positive macrophages containing bacillary bodies. The condition usually responds to broad-spectrum antibiotics.

Primary intestinal lymphoma usually arises in men under the age of 50 and may present with malabsorption. Malignant lymphoid cells infiltrate the lamina propria of the mucosa. Lymphadenopathy and hepatosplenomegaly are usually absent.

Disaccharidase (usually lactase) deficiency is most commonly secondary to infection, inflammation, celiac disease, or radiation enteritis; it is rarely inherited. Lactose cannot be broken down and the resulting osmotic load causes diarrhea. Morphology is normal and diagnosis is based on lactose challenge.

Endocrine System

DIRECTIONS: Each question below contains five suggested responses. Select the **one best** response to each question.

291. The most common etiologic factor in Cushing's syndrome is

(A) adrenal adenoma
(B) bilateral adrenal hyperplasia
(C) adrenal carcinoma
(D) ectopic adrenal tissue
(E) hypercorticism secondary to non-endocrine malignant tumors

292. An adult patient with seizure disorder controlled by phenytoin (Dilantin) is noted to have enlarged gingivae. Select the proper course of action below.

(A) No action is necessary because this is a drug effect
(B) No action is necessary because this is a physiologic response
(C) Schilling blood count should be performed
(D) Roentgenograms of the maxillae and mandible should be taken
(E) Biopsy with histologic examination should be performed

293. The combination of cystic bone lesions, precocious puberty, and patchy skin pigmentations is known as

(A) Albright's syndrome
(B) Letterer-Siwe disease
(C) Asherman's syndrome
(D) Morquio's disease
(E) Schaumann's disease

294. Follicular carcinoma of the thyroid may show all the following features EXCEPT

(A) vascular invasion and hematogenous metastasis
(B) multiple foci within the gland
(C) a clear cell variant that resembles renal carcinoma
(D) an insular type that is an aggressive form
(E) absence of ground-glass nuclei

295. The degree of hyperfunction in parathyroid glands affected by parathyroid adenoma depends on

(A) the type of cell involved
(B) the location of the adenomas in the neck or mediastinum
(C) the rate of growth of the adenoma
(D) the weight of parathyroid tissue
(E) serum calcium levels

296. A 42-year-old man complains of recently having to change his shoe size from 9 to 10½, and he also says that his hands and jaw are now larger. The disorder is most likely mediated through

(A) prolactin
(B) ACTH
(C) somatomedin
(D) antidiuretic hormone
(E) thyrotropin

297. The section of tissue shown in the photomicrograph below (taken under low power) was probably removed from a patient who has

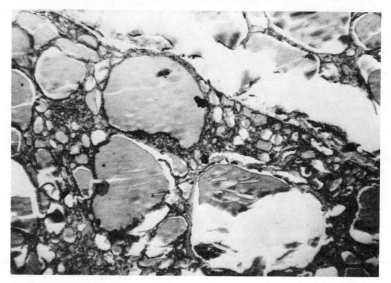

(A) a normal thyroid gland
(B) colloid storage goiter
(C) Graves' disease
(D) Riedel's struma
(E) Hashimoto's thyroiditis

298. All the following statements concerning thymomas are true EXCEPT

(A) they originate from epithelial cells
(B) they are most common in the anterosuperior mediastinum
(C) they are asymptomatic or cause local pressure effects
(D) neoplastic lymphocytes are a component
(E) most thymomas are benign

299. Secondary hyperparathyroidism may be caused by

(A) chronic renal insufficiency
(B) Hashimoto's thyroiditis
(C) pituitary hyperplasia
(D) alcoholic hepatitis
(E) acute pancreatitis

300. A perimenopausal woman complains of slight swallowing difficulty, fatigue, and a change in bowel habits. The photomicrograph below is of her thyroid gland. This disorder is

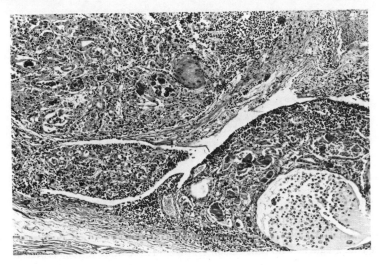

(A) subacute thyroiditis
(B) thyrotoxicosis
(C) autoimmune thyroiditis
(D) Riedel's thyroiditis
(E) conversion hysteria

---

301. Myelolipoma of the adrenal displays all the following characteristics EXCEPT

(A) origination in the inner zona fasciculata
(B) average diameter of 0.5 to 6 cm
(C) occasional intercostal and retroperitoneal occurrence
(D) rare inclusion of adrenocortical cells
(E) rare and late metastases

302. Primary hyperaldosteronism is associated with all the following features EXCEPT

(A) carcinoma
(B) adenoma
(C) muscle weakness
(D) expansion of intravascular volume
(E) edema

Questions 303-304

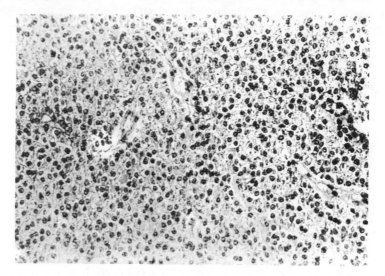

303. A young patient with renal insufficiency and bone lesions undergoes surgical neck exploration for investigation of a metabolic defect. The photomicrograph above indicates that the patient has

(A) malignant lymphoma
(B) chronic thyroiditis
(C) thyroid hyperplasia
(D) parathyroid hyperplasia
(E) Castelman's disease

304. These bone lesions represent

(A) lymphomatous dissemination
(B) osteomyelitis
(C) osteomalacia
(D) osteopetrosis
(E) osteochondrosis

305. A 49-year-old man who smokes two packs of cigarettes a day presents with a lung mass on x-ray and recent weight gain. Laboratory examination shows hyponatremia with hyperosmolar urine. The patient probably has

(A) renal failure
(B) pituitary failure
(C) Conn's syndrome
(D) cardiac failure
(E) inappropriate ADH

DIRECTIONS: Each question below contains four suggested responses of which **one or more** is correct. Select

A	if	**1, 2, and 3**	are correct
B	if	**1 and 3**	are correct
C	if	**2 and 4**	are correct
D	if	**4**	is correct
E	if	**1, 2, 3, and 4**	are correct

306. Diffuse toxic goiter is associated with

(1) localized dermatopathy
(2) cardiac manifestations
(3) proptosis
(4) HLA-DR5 genotype

307. Pheochromocytomas have been demonstrated in which of the following conditions?

(1) Multiple endocrine neoplasia, type IIb
(2) Von Hippel-Lindau syndrome
(3) Multiple endocrine neoplasia, type IIa
(4) Sturge-Weber syndrome

308. The parathyroid glands can be described in terms of anatomic or developmental characteristics that include

(1) embryonic development from the endodermal tissue of the third and fourth pharyngeal pouches
(2) the location of the superior glands normally at the lower border of the cricoid cartilage
(3) the location of the inferior glands sometimes in the superior mediastinum of the thorax
(4) a spatial relationship with the thyroid and a temporal developmental relationship with the thymus

DIRECTIONS: The group of questions below consists of four lettered headings followed by a set of numbered items. For each numbered item select

A	if the item is associated with	(A) **only**
B	if the item is associated with	(B) **only**
C	if the item is associated with	**both** (A) and (B)
D	if the item is associated with	**neither** (A) nor (B)

Each lettered heading may be used **once, more than once, or not at all.**

Questions 309-312

(A) Papillary carcinoma of the thyroid gland
(B) Medullary carcinoma of the thyroid gland
(C) Both
(D) Neither

309. Frequent follicular variants appear

310. Hematogenous metastasis is usual

311. Both sporadic and familial forms occur

312. Amyloid deposits are common

DIRECTIONS: The group of questions below consists of lettered headings followed by a set of numbered items. For each numbered item select the **one** lettered heading with which it is **most** closely associated. Each lettered heading may be used **once, more than once, or not at all.**

Questions 313-317

For each disorder listed, select the most appropriate feature or description.

(A) Panhypopituitarism in adults
(B) Cushing's syndrome in childhood
(C) Rare condition with very rare elaboration of hormones
(D) Postpartum pituitary necrosis
(E) Common cause of diabetes insipidus in children

313. Hand-Schüller-Christian disease

314. Sheehan's syndrome

315. Simmonds' disease

316. Pituitary carcinoma

317. Adrenal cortical carcinoma

Endocrine System

Answers

291. The answer is B. *(Braunwald, ed 11. pp 1760-1764.)* Cushing's syndrome may be the result of bilateral adrenal hyperplasia, adrenal neoplasia, or excessive use of adrenocorticotropic hormone or glucocorticoids. However, bilateral adrenal hyperplasia is the most common etiologic factor. The clinical manifestations of the syndrome, whether it is induced by ectopic ACTH (small-cell carcinoma of the lung), or exogenously, or endogenously by the adrenal, are similar. Levels of plasma and urinary cortisol and urinary 17-hydroxycorticoid are usually elevated.

292. The answer is C. *(Robbins, ed 4. p 821.)* There are multiple causes for enlarged gingivae, some of which are physiologic and transient and require no investigative or therapeutic measures. Among these is pregnancy, which under the stimulation of hormones produces a vascular proliferation that presents histology similar to that of pyogenic granuloma. Another physiologic response is that seen at puberty. Nutritional disorders such as vitamin C deficiency can also lead to enlarged gums. Phenytoin (Dilantin) has been known to cause enlargement of the gums in some patients. If the setting does not suggest a physiologic response, consideration should be given to leukemia, especially monocytic leukemia, which can present enlarged gums as the initial manifestation. Thus, a complete blood count, including a Schilling differential to enumerate the white cells, is indicated.

293. The answer is A. *(Anderson, ed 9. pp 1898-1900.)* The triad of cystic bone lesions, precocious puberty, and patchy brownish skin pigmentation is known as Albright's syndrome. The bone lesions are those of fibrous dysplasia and apparently result from abnormal activity by the bone-forming mesenchyma. Packing of the medullary cavity by fibrous tissue that contains trabeculae of poorly mineralized fibrous bone is seen in the lesions. Recent reports have described cases of fibrous dysplasia in both males and females who also have had a wide variety of endocrine abnormalities, including hyperthyroidism, acromegaly, and Cushing's syndrome.

294. The answer is B. *(Robbins, ed 4. pp 1234-1238.)* The four major histologic subtypes of thyroid carcinoma, in decreasing order of frequency, are papillary, follicular, medullary, and undifferentiated (anaplastic). Follicular carcinoma has a frequency of approximately 10 to 20 percent compared with papillary cancer at 60 to 70 percent. There are, of course, follicular variants of both papillary and medullary carcinoma, but these behave as papillary and medullary cancer, not as the follicular type. Other, much rarer variants of follicular cancer include the type resembling renal clear cell carcinoma and the insular type of thyroid cancer, which is an aggressive form of follicular carcinoma with a solid growth pattern. Vascular invasion and hematogenous metastasis are usual with follicular cancer, so that intrathyroidal foci from lymphatic spread would not occur, although they are very common with papillary cancer. Absence of ground-glass nuclei or well-formed papillae or psammoma bodies differentiates follicular from papillary carcinoma.

295. The answer is D. *(Robbins, ed 4. pp 1243-1244.)* Primary hyperparathyroidism can be caused by adenomas, chief cell hyperplasia, water–clear cell hyperplasia, or carcinoma. In the large majority of reported cases, single adenomas constitute the cause. Whether the histologic abnormality is hyperplasia or adenoma, a distinct correlation between the degree of hyperfunction and the weight of the parathyroid tissue has been demonstrated.

296. The answer is C. *(Henry, ed 17. pp 301-303. Robbins, ed 4. pp 1207-1210.)* The constellation of cartilaginous-periosteal soft tissue growth of the distal extremities (acromegaly) and growth of the skull and face bones is characteristic of hypersecretion of growth hormone (GH) from an anterior pituitary adenoma. GH modulates the production of hepatic somatomedin (sulfation factor). Somatomedins are small peptides that act on the target organs after being synthesized under the influence of growth hormone. They have insulin-like properties but are immunologically distinct from insulin. In addition to acral-skeletal expansion, patients with hyperpituitarism of the adult-onset variety (occurring after epiphyseal plate closure) have organomegaly, including increased size of the heart, kidneys, liver, and spleen. Cardiac failure is usually the mechanism of death.

297. The answer is B. *(Anderson, ed 9. pp 1546-1549.)* The histologic appearance of colloid storage goiter generally includes abnormally large, colloid-filled follicles compressing the intervening small or normal-sized follicles that contain very little colloid. The epithelium of the follicles is predominantly flat cuboidal, with occasional epithelial papillary structures protruding into the follicles. In primary hyperplasia with Graves' disease, the follicular epithelium is tall, with papillary infoldings and peripheral vacuolation of the colloid. Riedel's struma appears as a marked fibrous tissue replacement of the normal thyroid histology. In Hashimoto's thyroiditis, only remnants of thyroid follicles and epithelial cells are found in sheets of lymphocytes with germinal centers.

298. The answer is D. *(Robbins, ed 4. pp 1269-1271.)* Thymomas are tumors arising from thymic epithelial cells and form one of the most common mediastinal neoplasms, especially in the anterosuperior mediastinum. There is a scant or rich lymphocytic infiltrate of T cells, which are not neoplastic, although their size and prominent nucleoli may cause histologic confusion with lymphoma. About 90 percent of thymomas are benign and occur at a mean age of 50 years. They are very rare in children. They may be asymptomatic or cause pressure effects of dysphagia, dyspnea, or vena caval compression. Associated systemic disorders include myasthenia gravis, hematologic cytopenias, collagen vascular disease (lupus), and hypogammaglobulinemia. Malignant thymomas show infiltration and capsular invasion plus pleural implants or distant metastasis.

299. The answer is A. *(Robbins, ed 4. pp 1246-1247.)* Chronic hypocalcemia, whatever its origin, leads eventually to secondary hyperparathyroidism. Chronic renal failure is the most important cause, but secondary hyperparathyroidism also occurs in malabsorption syndromes, rickets, disseminated metastatic carcinoma, and multiple myeloma.

300. The answer is C. *(Robbins, ed 4. pp 1220-1222.)* Hashimoto's (autoimmune) thyroiditis is one of the conditions of chronic thyroiditis. It is not that uncommon in the United States. The stroma is permeated by a dense lymphoplasmacytic infiltrate with lymphoid follicles (germinal centers) that distorts and transforms thyroid follicles into collections of acidophilic cells (oncocytes, Hürthle-like cells). Not uncommonly, patients develop hypothyroidism as a result of follicle disruption, and the manifestations consist of fatigue, myxedema, cold intolerance, hair coarsening, and constipation. Whereas subacute (DeQuervain's) thyroiditis, Riedel's thyroiditis, and psychosomatic complaints may cause common symptoms, biopsy findings of these disorders are distinctly different from those of Hashimoto's disease.

301. The answer is E. *(Anderson, ed 9. pp 1605-1606.)* Myelolipoma is not clearly neoplastic; it is a circumscribed, yellow-red, tumor-like growth of bone marrow, composed microscopically of fat, red and white cell precursors, and megakaryocytes—a tissue resembling bone marrow surrounded by adrenal cortex. Origin appears to be in the inner zona fasciculata and it measures 0.5 to 6 cm in diameter, though it is occasionally larger. Extraadrenal myelolipomas may occur in the intercostal spaces and retroperitoneal or pelvic connective tissue. Rare adrenal myelolipomas have accompanied Cushing's syndrome and contained adrenocortical cells, but myelolipoma is usually incidental, without symptoms. It is a benign lesion, possibly representing mesenchymal rests.

302. The answer is E. *(Robbins, ed 4. pp 1259-1260.)* Edema is not a feature of primary hyperaldosteronism (Conn's syndrome), which is characterized by weakness, hypertension, polydipsia, and polyuria. The underlying physiologic abnormalities include alkaline urine, an elevated level of serum sodium, hypokalemic alkalosis, and excessive potassium loss by the kidneys. The level of serum aldosterone is elevated; that of plasma renin is suppressed. The elevated level of serum sodium causes expansion of the intravascular volume. A single adenoma has been described as the causative factor of primary hyperaldosteronism in the majority of patients, and carcinoma, multiple adenomas, and cortical hyperplasia have been cited occasionally as causes of this syndrome.

303. The answer is D. *(Robbins, ed 4. pp 1245-1247.)* Hypocalcemia resulting from any chronic cause may lead to hyperparathyroidism. The mechanism of hypocalcemia in chronic renal failure is thought to be related to phosphate retention. Sustained parathormone release results from the chronic hypocalcemia. The parathyroid hyperplasia under these circumstances may involve one, two, three, or all four parathyroid glands in the form of chief cell hyperplasia, frequently with scattered nests of eosinophilic, oxyphilic cells (oncocytes). There is an accompanying replacement of the intraglandular fat by the hyperplasia. Surgical extirpation is the treatment of choice.

304. The answer is C. *(Robbins, ed 4. pp 1243-1246.)* Primary hyperparathyroidism (HPT), as in parathyroid adenoma, leads to more extensive bone disease than is found in secondary hyperparathyroidism, as in chronic renal failure. Calcium levels are generally higher in the primary form of the disease than in the secondary form, in which calcium levels are low or low-normal; accordingly, the bone lesions are more severe in primary HPT, and through a process of bone resorption and fibrous replacement, cystic spaces result (osteitis fibrosa cystica). Repeated hemorrhages may occur in these focal lesions, with the formation of reactive granulomas (brown tumors). This is a rare event, since hypercalcemia is actively sought out and is treated early in most medical centers. The bone lesions in secondary hyperparathyroidism are of a milder degree and consist basically of a demineralization process (osteomalacia); this can be recognized as too much osteoid without appropriate mineralization. Osteoporosis involves a loss of bone, with osteoid-mineralization reduction being proportionately reduced. Osteopetrosis (Albers-Schönberg disease, or marble bone disease) is an inherited bone disease characterized by bony sclerosis and excess bone growths with loss of marrow spaces.

305. The answer is E. *(Robbins, ed 4. p 801.)* The syndrome of inappropriate antidiuretic hormone (SIADH) is an important cause of dilutional hyponatremia that has been identified in tumors of the thymus gland, malignant lymphoma, and pancreatic neoplasms. It occurs predominantly, however, as a result of ectopic secretion of ADH by oat cell carcinomas of the lung. Since the tumor cells per se are autonomously producing ADH, there is no feedback inhibition from the hypothalamic osmoreceptors, and the persistent ADH effect on the renal tubules causes water retention even with concentrated urine. Hence the term *inappropriate ADH* arises. Laboratory findings of the syndrome include low plasma sodium levels (dilutional hyponatremia), low plasma osmolality, and high urine osmolality caused by disproportionate solute excretion without water.

306. The answer is A (1, 2, 3). *(Robbins, ed 4. pp 1217-1218, 1224-1226.)* Graves' disease is one of the three most common disorders associated with hyperthyroidism—the other two being toxic multinodular goiter and toxic adenoma. The syndrome of Graves' disease consists of thyrotoxicosis caused by a hyperfunctioning diffuse hyperplastic goiter accompanied by ophthalmopathy and dermatopathy, or localized "myxedema," present in only 10 to 15 percent of cases. Localized, edematous thickened skin is noted over the dorsal legs or feet. Cardiac manifestations—tachycardia, palpitations, cardiomegaly, and occasional arrhythmias—are among the earliest and most consistent features. Protrusion of the globe distinguishes Graves' disease from other forms of thyrotoxicosis and is secondary to immunoinflammatory changes in retroorbital tissues. Marked thickening of extraocular muscles is easily recognized on CT scan and is an important diagnostic sign. HLA-DR5 genotype is associated with Hashimoto's thyroiditis, whereas diffuse toxic goiter is associated with HLA-DR3 genotype.

307. The answer is A (1, 2, 3). *(Robbins, ed 4. pp 1262-1265.)* Multiple endocrine neoplasia (MEN, or adenomatosis) syndromes are an interesting collection of predominantly benign tumors of the endocrine system that are inheritable in an incompletely penetrating autosomal dominant manner. MEN type I consists of functioning adenomas of the pituitary, pancreas, parathyroid, and adrenal glands with peptic ulcers. Type II (medullary thyroid carcinoma) disorders include pheochromocytomas and parathyroid adenomas and are subclassified as type "a" (no neuromas) and type "b" (lip and oral neuromas). Patients with von Hippel-Lindau syndrome may also have pheochromocytomas, in addition to adrenal myelolipomas, epididymal cystadenomas, and cerebellar hemangioblastomas. Patients with Sturge-Weber syndrome (oculomeningeal nevus flammens) have not been noted to have pheochromocytomas.

308. The answer is E (all). *(Anderson, ed 9. p 1570.)* The parathyroid glands develop from the endodermal tissue of the dorsal diverticula of the third and fourth pharyngeal pouches and usually consist of four flattened, encapsulated, oval bodies that lie against the dorsum of the thyroid gland. The superior glands, derived from the fourth pharyngeal pouches, have an anatomic position that is more constant than that of the inferior pair. The inferior parathyroids, because they develop and move caudally with the thymus, sometimes become located below the thyroid level, and the inconstant location of these parathyroids is an important factor to consider in the search for pathologic parathyroid tissue during autopsy or surgery.

309-312. The answers are: 309-A, 310-D, 311-B, 312-B. *(Robbins, ed 4. pp 1233-1240.)* Papillary carcinoma is the most common type of thyroid cancer and has the best prognosis, although lymphatic invasion is usual, which accounts for both the common metastasis to cervical lymph nodes and for the multifocal intrathyroidal spread. About 50 percent of all papillary thyroid carcinomas show follicular differentiation (follicular variants), but their biologic behavior is that of papillary carcinoma with very slow growth and long survival. Psammoma bodies are found in about 40 percent of papillary tumors (stippled calcification on x-ray) and nuclei often show characteristic clearing or ground-glass appearance. Papillary carcinoma has been related to irradiation of head and neck in early life.

Hematogenous metastasis to brain, bone, or lungs is the usual mode of spread of follicular carcinoma, which, when well differentiated, may be confused with follicular adenoma except for invasion of blood vessels or capsule.

Medullary carcinoma of the thyroid (MCT) originates from the parafollicular C cells. It occurs in both sporadic and familial forms; the latter occurs before 30 years of age and is associated with pheochromocytomas and parathyroid hyperplasia or adenoma (Sipple's syndrome, MEN IIa). The parafollicular cells secrete calcitonin and carcinoembryonic antigen and, occasionally, ACTH, prostaglandin, serotonin, or bradykinin. Measurements of elevated serum calcitonin are useful both in diagnosis and prognosis, especially in familial settings, where family members should be screened for elevated serum levels. Follicular variants are rare but amyloid stromal deposits are frequent in MCT, which has an indolent or aggressive course.

313-317. The answers are: 313-E, 314-D, 315-A, 316-C, 317-B. *(Anderson, ed 9. pp 1526-1527, 1529, 1599-1605.)* Panhypopituitarism results from destruction of at least 75 percent of the anterior pituitary. This destruction usually is caused by tumors (e.g., metastatic carcinoma of the breast or lung) and infarction, but destruction can also be caused by inflammatory disorders, abscesses, granulomas (giant-cell granulomas of older women), and histiocytic infiltrates. *Simmonds' disease*— the eponym for the classic clinical syndrome caused by panhypopituitarism in the adult—involves insufficiency of the gonads, thyroid, and adrenals and is secondary to the absence of stimulation by the respective trophic hormones.

Sheehan's syndrome consists of symptoms of pituitary failure that occur as the result of infarction of the pituitary because of postpartum hemorrhage or other types of massive hemorrhage. In Sheehan's syndrome the pituitary infarction frequently occurs in the presence of intravascular coagulopathy of pregnancy.

Hand-Schüller-Christian disease (HSC) features histiocytic infiltrates in the pituitary and xanthomatous deposits in the skull and dura. Because the infundibular portion of the pituitary may be involved in HSC, the disease may cause diabetes insipidus in children as the pituitary is subjected to bony encasement with destruction of the nerve tracts in the neurohypophysis.

Before the age of 10, Cushing's syndrome is probably most often related to adrenal carcinoma, a tumor present in at least 50 percent of cases, while most of the remaining cases are associated with adrenocortical hyperplasia. After the age of 10, zona fasciculata hyperplasia accounts for approximately 70 percent of cases. In the adult, adrenocortical carcinoma is responsible for only 10 percent of the cases of Cushing's syndrome. Adrenal carcinomas are differentiated from adenomas by capsular or vascular invasion and metastasis.

Primary carcinoma of the anterior pituitary is not only rare but is rather undifferentiated, so that the cell type cannot be identified. However, most cases are of chromophobe origin; therefore, hormonal elaboration is very rare. It is difficult to differentiate the carcinoma from an adenoma and very local invasion is also unreliable; thus, metastasis is the only valid criterion of malignancy.

Genitourinary System

DIRECTIONS: Each question below contains five suggested responses. Select the **one best** response to each question.

318. The photomicrograph below depicts a biopsy of the uterine cervix that was done following an abnormal Pap smear report. This histologic section shows

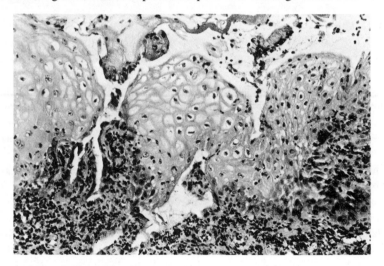

(A) condyloma acuminatum
(B) carcinoma in situ
(C) dysplasia
(D) cervical intraepithelial neoplasia
(E) squamous metaplasia

319. A middle-aged man comes to you with the single presenting symptom of occasional hematuria of very recent onset. The most probable cause is

(A) acute pyelonephritis
(B) nephroblastoma
(C) renal cell carcinoma
(D) mesoblastic nephroma
(E) renal pelvic urothelial tumor

320. All the following statements are true of urinary calculi EXCEPT that

(A) they are more common in males than in females
(B) they are bilateral in 40 percent of cases
(C) they are radiopaque in about 90 percent of cases
(D) they may be associated with *Pseudomonas* infections
(E) the incidence is increased in leukemia

321. A linear pattern of immunoglobulin deposition along the glomerular basement membrane that can be demonstrated by immunofluorescence is typical of

(A) lupus nephritis
(B) diabetic glomerulopathy
(C) Goodpasture's syndrome
(D) Goldblatt's kidney
(E) renal vein thrombosis

322. What is the correct treatment for a patient who has hypertension secondary to unilateral renal artery stenosis when the contralateral kidney shows severe arteriolonephrosclerosis?

(A) Ureteral reimplantation
(B) Removal of the kidney supplied by the stenotic artery
(C) Repair of the renal artery stenosis and ipsilateral nephrectomy
(D) Repair of the renal artery stenosis and contralateral nephrectomy
(E) Nonsurgical management

323. Marked glomerular basement membrane thickening, as shown in the photomicrograph below, may be seen in all the following conditions EXCEPT

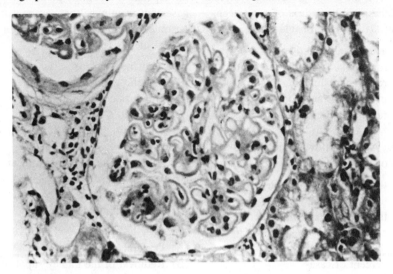

(A) lupus nephritis
(B) membranous glomerulonephritis
(C) diabetes mellitus
(D) acute pyelonephritis
(E) renal vein thrombosis

324. The gross appearance of the kidney illustrated (right) is most compatible with which of the following conditions?

(A) Cystic renal dysplasia
(B) Acute pyelonephritis
(C) Chronic pyelonephritis
(D) Acute glomerulonephritis
(E) Chronic glomerulonephritis

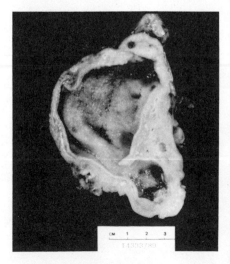

325. An adult medical laboratory technician recovering from hepatitis B develops hematuria, proteinuria, and red cell casts in the urine. Which of the following would best describe the changes occurring within the kidney in this patient?

(A) Plasma cell interstitial nephritis
(B) IgG linear fluorescence along the glomerular basement membrane
(C) Granular deposits of antibodies in the glomerular basement membrane
(D) Diffuse glomerular basement membrane thickening by subepithelial immune deposits
(E) Nodular hyaline glomerulosclerosis

326. All the following characteristics are associated with the disorder depicted in the photograph below EXCEPT

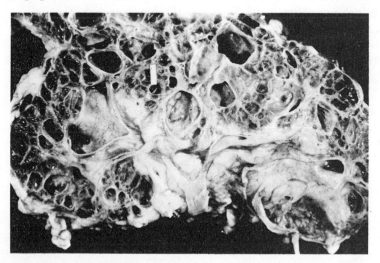

(A) massive unilateral enlargement
(B) autosomal dominance in adults
(C) autosomal recessive in childhood
(D) hepatic cysts in childhood form
(E) possible association with berry aneurysms

327. A sexually active adult male who has had a negative evaluation for gonococcus infection and who complains of persistent dysuria but no other symptoms should be considered to have

(A) prostatic hypertrophy
(B) epididymitis
(C) orchitis
(D) nonspecific urethritis
(E) renal stones

328. A 46-year-old woman undergoes an abdominal hysterectomy for a "fibroid" uterus. The surgeon requests a frozen section on the tumor, which is deferred because of the lesion's degree of cellularity. Which of the following criteria will be used by the pathologist in determining benignancy versus malignancy in permanent sections?

(A) Mitotic rate
(B) Cell pleomorphism
(C) Cell necrosis
(D) Nucleocytoplasmic (NC) ratio
(E) Tumor size

329. Which of the following is sufficiently different from the others to be discriminated by histologic examination only?

(A) Bowen's disease
(B) Squamous cell carcinoma in situ
(C) Erythroplasia of Queyrat
(D) Bowenoid papulosis
(E) Human papilloma virus (HPV) condyloma

330. A 23-year-old woman with an abnormal Pap smear undergoes a cervical biopsy. The results are read as "CIN-2." What is the meaning of this report?

(A) Cervical carcinoma, grade II
(B) Cervical carcinoma, stage II
(C) Cervical inflammation; repeat in 2 months
(D) Carcinoma in situ
(E) Moderate dysplasia

331. The photomicrograph below is of a section from a testis removed from the inguinal region of a man aged 25. Which of the following statements is true regarding the condition illustrated?

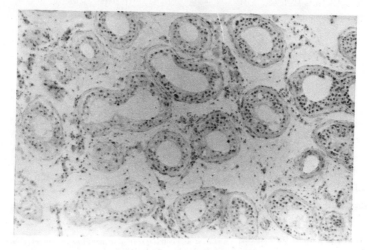

(A) It occurs in 5 percent of the adult male population
(B) Teratoma is the most common malignancy to arise
(C) Risk of associated malignancy is reduced by orchiopexy
(D) There is increased risk of malignancy in the contralateral testis
(E) Both Leydig and Sertoli cells are reduced in number

332. The condition shown in the photomicrograph, malacoplakia of the urinary bladder, is considered to be associated with

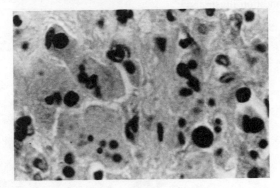

(A) tuberculosis
(B) urothelial carcinoma
(C) schistosomiasis
(D) staphylococcal infections
(E) defects in phagocytosis

333. A woman harboring endometrial adenocarcinoma nearly always has antecedent

(A) obesity
(B) diabetes mellitus
(C) endometrial polyps
(D) endometrial hyperplasia
(E) systemic hypertension

334. The ovarian lesion in the photomicrograph below is

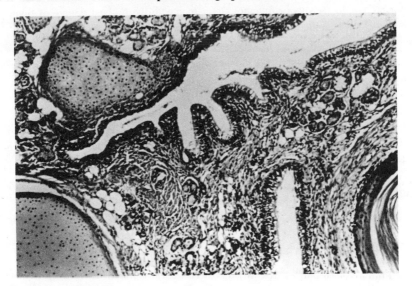

(A) chronic salpingitis
(B) an ectopic pregnancy
(C) a granulosa cell tumor
(D) a cystic teratoma
(E) metastatic squamous cell carcinoma

---

335. A 10-year-old boy has a bout of ordinary upper respiratory infection followed within 36 hours by an episode of hematuria. There are no joint symptoms, gastrointestinal symptoms, petechiae, or rashes. To confirm the suspicion of Berger's disease, which of the following is indicated?

(A) Examination of urinary sediment
(B) Renal scan
(C) Renal biopsy immunofluorescence
(D) Creatinine clearance
(E) Intravenous pyelogram

336. Vaginal adenosis precedes the development of which of the following?

(A) Cervical carcinoma
(B) Condyloma acuminatum
(C) Clear cell carcinoma
(D) Carcinoma of the endometrium
(E) Squamous carcinoma of the vagina

337. The majority of malignant tumors of the ovary take their origin from

(A) surface epithelium
(B) urogenital stem cells
(C) ovarian germ cells
(D) stromal cells
(E) hilar cells

338. Ovarian cystadenomas or cystadenocarcinomas (serous or mucinous)

(A) always produce androgens
(B) seldom are bilateral
(C) can be papillary
(D) usually occur during pregnancy
(E) are extremely rare

339. Metastatic, mucin-producing, signet-ring cancer cells in the ovary most frequently come from

(A) gastrointestinal carcinoma
(B) endometrial carcinoma
(C) malignant melanoma
(D) astrocytoma
(E) histiocytic lymphoma

340. Primary germ cell tumors of the testis occur predominantly in the younger male with the exception of

(A) embryonal carcinoma
(B) spermatocytic seminoma
(C) polyembryoma
(D) choriocarcinoma
(E) teratocarcinoma

341. In the list below the ovarian tumor with the highest degree of bilateral involvement is

(A) endometrioid carcinoma
(B) serous cystadenoma
(C) mucinous cystadenoma
(D) mucinous cystadenocarcinoma
(E) serous cystadenocarcinoma

342. A small, palpable, well-circumscribed nodule in the epididymis is most likely to be

(A) androblastoma
(B) tuberculous granuloma
(C) carcinoma
(D) adenomatoid tumor
(E) adrenocortical rest

343. Which of the following genera is most responsible for venereal disease in women in the United States?

(A) *Calymmatobacterium*
(B) *Campylobacter*
(C) *Chlamydia*
(D) *Neisseria*
(E) *Haemophilus*

344. The cells in the photomicrograph below were the predominant type in a Papanicolaou stained smear of the lateral vaginal wall from a 66-year-old woman. The cell pattern shows a predominance of

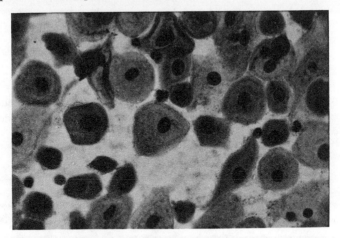

(A) superficial squamous cells
(B) intermediate squamous cells
(C) parabasal squamous cells
(D) malignant squamous cells
(E) histiocytes

345. All the following statements are true regarding transitional cell carcinoma of the bladder EXCEPT that

(A) it is more common in men than in women
(B) it is associated with infection by *Schistosoma haematobium*
(C) it is associated with cigarette smoking
(D) it shows increased incidence in aniline dye workers
(E) it tends to recur after excision, regardless of grade

DIRECTIONS: Each question below contains four suggested responses of which **one or more** is correct. Select

A	if	**1, 2, and 3**	are correct
B	if	**1 and 3**	are correct
C	if	**2 and 4**	are correct
D	if	**4**	is correct
E	if	**1, 2, 3, and 4**	are correct

346. A patient being investigated for hematuria and proteinuria has a renal biopsy that shows changes in the glomeruli as depicted below. Which of the following diseases can be associated with changes seen in this biopsy?

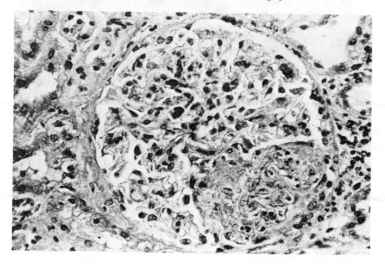

(1) Bacterial endocarditis
(2) Anaphylactoid purpura
(3) Systemic lupus erythematosus
(4) Hereditary nephritis (Alport's syndrome)

347. Acute poststreptococcal glomerulonephritis usually

(1) affects children
(2) follows a streptococcal infection by more than 6 months
(3) is accompanied by decreased serum complement
(4) leads to chronic renal failure

348. Diseases of the urinary tract occurring with increased frequency in patients with diabetes mellitus include

(1) nephrotic syndrome
(2) atherosclerosis of the renal artery
(3) renal papillary necrosis
(4) acute pyelonephritis

349. The photomicrograph below shows evidence of glomerular fibrin deposition. This histopathology is a supplemental finding in a 2-year-old child who has a history of abdominal pain and bloody diarrhea, followed by acute glomerulonephritis, Coombs'-negative severe hemolytic anemia, and renal failure. The likely diagnoses might include

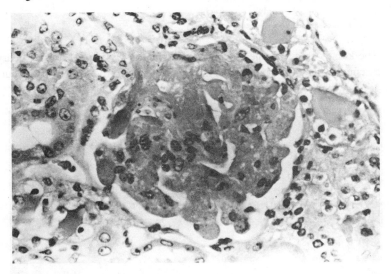

(1) lupus erythematosus
(2) acute poststreptococcal glomerulonephritis
(3) lipoid nephrosis
(4) hemolytic-uremic syndrome

---

350. True statements concerning the hemolytic-uremic syndrome (HUS) in young children include that

(1) endothelial injury is an initiating pathologic event
(2) prior infection with *E. coli* is common
(3) hypertension exists in about half the patients
(4) involvement of the CNS is a dominant feature

SUMMARY OF DIRECTIONS

A	B	C	D	E
1, 2, 3 only	1, 3 only	2, 4 only	4 only	All are correct

351. The kidney shown in the photomicrograph below is affected by a primary renal carcinoma that has originated in the upper pole. Correct statements about renal primary carcinoma include that

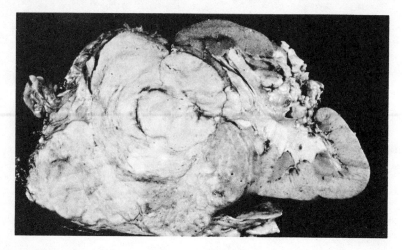

(1) in gross examination, the lesions are spherical masses of tissue that may be bright yellow
(2) in microscopic evaluation, the cellular character is squamous or papillary
(3) these tumors characteristically invade the renal veins
(4) the neoplastic tissue probably secretes adrenocorticotropic hormone

352. Components of diabetic glomerulopathy include

(1) diffuse glomerulosclerosis
(2) nodular glomerulosclerosis
(3) thickening of capillary basement membranes
(4) mesangial proliferation

353. The nephrotic syndrome is associated with which of the following renal disorders?

(1) Membranous glomerulonephritis
(2) Lipoid nephrosis
(3) Membranoproliferative glomerulonephritis
(4) Acute tubular necrosis

354. Which of the following renal diseases may cause hypertension?

(1) Renal artery arteriosclerosis
(2) Fibromuscular dysplasia of the renal artery
(3) Hydronephrosis
(4) Pyelonephritis

355. Renal diseases in which fibrin thrombi play a prominent role include

(1) lipoid nephrosis
(2) membranous glomerulopathy
(3) diabetes mellitus
(4) anaphylactoid purpura (Henoch-Schönlein purpura)

356. Risk factors for squamous carcinoma of the cervix include

(1) early sexual activity
(2) multiple sexual partners
(3) human papilloma virus types 16/18
(4) herpes simplex virus type 2

357. Carcinoma of the prostate tends to

(1) be adenocarcinoma
(2) arise in the posterior lobe
(3) cause elevation of serum acid phosphatase
(4) be estrogen-dependent

358. An elderly man experiences nocturnal dysuria, polyuria, and frequency. As a result of the process most likely to cause these symptoms at an advanced age, which of the following effects can be predicted?

(1) Hemorrhagic cystitis
(2) Septicemia
(3) Bladder trabeculation
(4) Bladder dilatation

359. A young woman with lower pelvic pain, menometrorrhagia, and a negative beta-HcG test undergoes uterine dilatation and curettage. The pathology report on the endometrial curettings states, "Compatible with decidualized gestational hyperplasia, no chorionic villi present." The next step or steps would be to

(1) repeat the beta-HcG test
(2) discharge the patient
(3) consider ectopic pregnancy
(4) consider appendicitis

SUMMARY OF DIRECTIONS

A	B	C	D	E
1, 2, 3 only	1, 3 only	2, 4 only	4 only	All are correct

360. An 18-month-old infant is evaluated for generalized tissue edema and ascites. Urinalysis shows numerous hyaline casts and lipid droplets. Total plasma protein and albumin are markedly decreased, whereas total lipids are increased. A light micrograph of a renal biopsy glomerulus is shown below. Statements applicable to this disorder include that

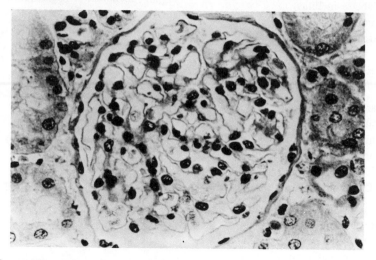

(1) the problem is hepatic, not renal
(2) electron microscopy is diagnostic
(3) light microscopy is diagnostic
(4) exacerbations are not uncommon

361. A female patient is being treated with penicillin for acute salpingitis and pelvic inflammatory disease without benefit. Which of the following organisms should now be considered in the differential diagnosis?

(1) *Bacteroides* species
(2) *Neisseria gonorrhoeae*
(3) *Chlamydia trachomatis*
(4) Adenoviruses

362. Cystic hyperplasia of the endometrium

(1) often occurs at or just before menopause
(2) occurs in association with increased estrogen administration or production
(3) usually results in excessive uterine bleeding
(4) is associated with secretory cells lining the cystically dilated glands

363. Neoplasms that have been reported in increased incidence in homosexual men include

(1) cloacogenic carcinoma
(2) malignant lymphoma
(3) Kaposi's sarcoma
(4) Bowen's disease

364. A major role in the exclusion of albumin from the ultrafiltrate in the normal human glomerulus is played by

(1) sodium-potassium ATPase
(2) parietal epithelium
(3) endothelial fenestrations
(4) proteoglycans

365. A significant role in vascular permeability, particularly in the renal glomerulus, is played by

(1) desmin
(2) fibronectin
(3) podocytes
(4) polyanions

SUMMARY OF DIRECTIONS

A	B	C	D	E
1, 2, 3 only	1, 3 only	2, 4 only	4 only	All are correct

366. Common outcomes of the uterine abnormality illustrated below include

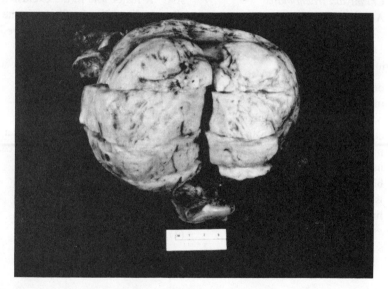

(1) cystic degeneration
(2) calcification
(3) rapid enlargement during pregnancy
(4) accelerated growth after menopause

---

367. A granulosa cell tumor of the ovary may produce excess estrogen and cause

(1) menstrual irregularities
(2) endometrial hyperplasia
(3) precocious puberty
(4) uterine enlargement

368. Ascites and pleural effusion have been detected in a woman with a primary ovarian neoplasm. These findings

(1) mean that the tumor has metastasized and is thus inoperable
(2) are strong presumptive evidence that a granulosa cell tumor is present in an ovary
(3) indicate that the patient should receive intrapleural administration of methotrexate and actinomycin D
(4) may occur with a benign ovarian fibroma

369. Which of the following at the present time can be considered to be conclusive evidence of coitus if found in vaginal fluid?

(1) Alkaline phosphatase
(2) Acid phosphatase
(3) Prostatic acid phosphatase
(4) p30

370. Mumps orchitis generally

(1) is bilateral
(2) results in sterility
(3) occurs simultaneously with parotid swelling
(4) occurs in adults

371. The photomicrograph below shows an abnormal renal tubular epithelial cell in a urinary specimen from a very ill renal transplant patient. The disease diagnosed is associated with

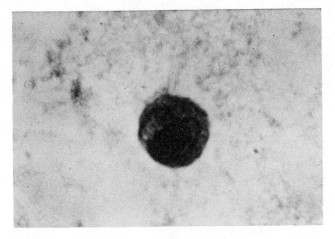

(1) interstitial pneumonitis
(2) hepatitis
(3) a herpesvirus
(4) gastrointestinal ulcers

372. Primary malignant neoplasms of the vagina include

(1) sarcoma botryoides
(2) clear cell carcinoma
(3) squamous carcinoma
(4) vaginal adenosis

373. The photomicrograph below shows a section through a testis removed from a 45-year-old man with acute scrotal pain. True statements regarding this condition include that

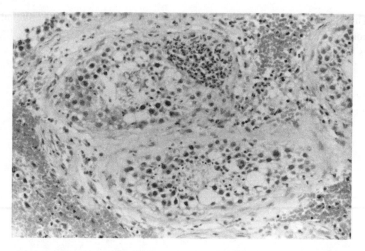

(1) infection is usually by the hematogenous route
(2) sterility is a common complication
(3) the epididymis is usually spared
(4) *Chlamydia trachomatis* is a common pathogen

DIRECTIONS: Each group of questions below consists of lettered headings followed by a set of numbered items. For each numbered item select the **one** lettered heading with which it is **most** closely associated. Each lettered heading may be used **once, more than once, or not at all.**

Questions 374-376

Match the renal disorders with the pathologic findings with which they are most likely to be associated.

(A) Hyalinized glomeruli
(B) Splitting of the glomerular basement membranes
(C) Diffuse thickening of capillary walls
(D) Glomerular hypercellularity and leukocytes
(E) Glomerular epithelial crescents

374. Membranoproliferative glomerulonephritis

375. Membranous glomerulonephritis

376. Goodpasture's syndrome

Questions 377-379

Choose the disease in which each pathologic finding is most characteristic.

(A) Malignant hypertension
(B) Systemic lupus erythematosus
(C) Chronic thyroiditis
(D) Addison's disease
(E) Diabetic nephropathy

377. Hyperplastic arteriolar nephrosclerosis

378. Nodular or intercapillary glomerulosclerosis

379. Necrotizing papillitis

DIRECTIONS: The groups of questions below consist of four lettered headings followed by a set of numbered items. For each numbered item select

A	if the item is associated with	(A) **only**
B	if the item is associated with	(B) **only**
C	if the item is associated with	**both** (A) and (B)
D	if the item is associated with	**neither** (A) nor (B)

Each lettered heading may be used **once, more than once, or not at all.**

Questions 380-384

(A) Choriocarcinoma
(B) Hydatidiform mole
(C) Both
(D) Neither

380. Production of alpha-fetoprotein (AFP)

381. Malignancy of trophoblastic cells

382. Occurrence in 1 in 2000 pregnancies in U.S.

383. Primary germ cell tumor of testis

384. Considerable elevation in titers of human chorionic gonadotropin (HCG)

Questions 385-388

(A) Minimal change disease (lipoid nephrosis)
(B) Focal segmental glomerulosclerosis
(C) Both
(D) Neither

385. Association with nephrotic syndrome

386. Association with AIDS

387. Very good response to steroid therapy

388. Deposition of IgM and C3

Genitourinary System
Answers

318. The answer is A. *(Richart, Cancer 60:1951-1959, 1987. Robbins, ed 4. pp 1135, 1142-1143.)* Cervical condylomata, particularly flat condylomata, although benign are considered to be precursors of cervical intraepithelial neoplasia (CIN), which comprises both dysplasia and carcinoma in situ (CIS). Histologically, these condylomata consist of connective tissue stroma covered by hyperplastic epithelium with prominent perinuclear cytoplasmic vacuolization (koilocytosis). Koilocytotic cells are characteristic of human papilloma virus (HPV) infection. More than 50 genotypes of HPV are known at present, and condylomata acuminata are associated with types 6/11 while HPV types 16/18 are usually present in CIN. Following an abnormal Pap smear report suggesting condyloma, CIN, or possible invasive carcinoma, work-up of the patient should include colposcopy, multiple cervical punch biopsies, and endocervical curettage to distinguish patients who have invasive cancer, CIN, or flat condylomata.

319. The answer is E. *(Robbins, ed 4. p 1078.)* A middle-aged patient is highly unlikely to have either of the predominantly childhood tumors nephroblastoma (Wilms' tumor) or mesoblastic nephroma (benign hamartoma). Mesoblastic nephroma, which may be seen in the first year of life, has caused difficulty in differential diagnosis from Wilms' tumor in children. Acute pyelonephritis features signs of acute infection with flank pain, pyuria, fever, and a high bacterial colony count in urine. Renal cell carcinoma is unlikely to cause hematuria until far advanced with invasion of the collecting system. Urothelial renal pelvic tumors cause hematuria early, even when quite small. They form 5 to 10 percent of primary renal tumors and range from apparently benign papillomas to papillary or anaplastic carcinomas. There may be multicentric involvement of ureters or bladder. Diagnosis is by x-ray and cytologic examination of at least three voided urine specimens; malignant cells are not found if the ureter is obstructed by tumor, or if the cells are degenerate or mildly atypical, as in papilloma. Prognosis is not very good for high-grade infiltrating tumors and is very poor for the squamous cell variant (about 15 percent of pelvic tumors); therefore, early diagnosis is paramount.

320. The answer is B. *(Robbins, ed 4. pp 1073-1074).* Urinary calculi are a common problem and may arise at any level of the urinary tract, but mainly in the kidney. They are more common in males and most patients are over 30 years of age. Urinary calculi are unilateral in 80 percent of cases, and 90 percent are radiopaque since most contain calcium oxalate or calcium phosphate. Other constituents include magnesium ammonium phosphate, cystine, and uric acid. Urate stones are radiolucent and are increased in hyperuricemia due to gout and in conditions with rapid cell turnover such as leukemia. Urea-splitting organisms such as *Pseudomonas* predispose to calculi.

321. The answer is C. *(Robbins, ed 4. pp 1031-1032.)* In Goodpasture's syndrome, circulating antibodies reactive with the glomerular basement membrane will bind in a linear pattern along the entire length of the glomerular basement membrane, which is their specific antigen. IgG is deposited in the basement membrane, along with complement. There are focal interruptions of the glomerular basement membrane as well, along with deposits of fibrin, as seen with electron microscopy.

322. The answer is D. *(Robbins, ed 4. pp 1068-1069.)* In a patient with a surgically correctable lesion of the renal artery, the corresponding kidney, which is potentially the less damaged one, should be saved. The contralateral kidney may be severely affected with arteriolonephrosclerosis and could perpetuate the hypertension if not removed. In a patient with parenchymal renal disease leading to hypertension, such as pyelonephritis, removal of the affected kidney may relieve the hypertension.

323. The answer is D. *(Robbins, ed 4. pp 198-200, 1043.)* The thickening of the basement membrane in systemic lupus erythematosus and membranous glomerulonephritis is thought to result from deposition of immune complexes. The pathogenesis of this same lesion in diabetes mellitus and renal vein thrombosis is unknown. Electron-dense deposits are classically seen in a subendothelial position on the glomerular basement membrane but may be subepithelial as well in some cases.

324. The answer is C. *(Robbins, ed 4. pp 1019, 1042-1043, 1055-1057.)* The kidney illustrated is typical of chronic pyelonephritis with dilatation of the renal pelvis, clubbing of the calyces, and irregular reduction in parenchymal mass. Chronic pyelonephritis is an asymmetric, irregularly scarring process that may be unilateral or bilateral. Microscopically, there is atrophy and dilatation of tubules with colloid in some tubules. Chronic inflammation and fibrosis occur in the cortex and medulla. Chronic glomerulonephritis causes bilateral, symmetrically shrunken and scarred kidneys. Histologic changes depend on the stage of the disease. Cystic dysplasia is characterized by undifferentiated mesenchyme and immature cartilage and collecting ductules.

325. The answer is C. *(Robbins, ed 4. pp 1024-1036.)* Glomerular injury caused by circulating antigen-antibody complexes is a secondary effect from a nonprimary renal source. Numerous clinical examples exist of a serum sickness–like nephritis as a consequence of systemic infection, with classical clinical models such as syphilis, hepatitis B, malaria, and bacterial endocarditis leading to renal disease. Immune complexes to antigens from any of these sources are circulating within the vascular system and become entrapped within the filtration system of the glomerular basement membranes. This can be seen as granular bumpy deposits by immunofluorescence within the basement membranes of the glomeruli. Linear fluorescence, on the other hand, is seen in primary antiglomerular basement membrane disease, wherein antibodies are directed against the glomerular basement membrane itself. Plasma cell interstitial nephritis is seen in immunologic rejection of transplanted kidneys. Nodular glomerulosclerosis is an effect of diabetes mellitus. The presence of red blood cell casts in the urine nearly always indicates that there has been glomerular injury, but is not specific for any given cause. Glomerular basement membrane thickening caused by subepithelial immune deposits is seen in membranous glomerulonephritis. While the morphology of membranous glomerulonephritis is different from that of nephritis caused by circulating antigen-antibody complexes (immune complexes), there are similarities in the pathogenesis in that both disorders may be a consequence of or in association with infections such as hepatitis B, syphilis, and malaria. Other causes for membranous glomerulonephritis include reactions to penicillamine, gold, and certain malignancies such as malignant melanoma.

326. The answer is A. *(Robbins, ed 4. pp 1018-1021.)* Polycystic kidney disease is a serious renal disorder that is inherited in two forms. The adult form is autosomal dominant with high penetrance of nearly 100 percent involvement of progeny who live to be older. The childhood polycystic form is autosomal recessive in inheritance. In the adult form one-third of the patients have cysts within the liver, while nearly all the childhood cases have hepatic cysts. Congenital hepatic fibrosis is associated with childhood polycystic kidney disease. In the adult form bilateral renal involvement is nearly invariable. One-third of patients with the adult form of polycystic kidney disease succumb to renal failure, while death occurs in another third as a consequence of hypertension.

327. The answer is D. *(Robbins, ed 4. pp 1095-1096.)* Nonspecific urethritis may actually be the most common cause of dysuria in sexually active males, although gonorrhea should always be excluded by laboratory examination. Causes of nonspecific urethritis include some bacteria, such as *Escherichia coli* and streptococci, but recent evidence implicates chlamydiae of the TRIC group as being perhaps the most common offending agents. The organism may take up residence in the prostate, producing chronic and active prostatitis. Prostatic hypertrophy, epididymitis, orchitis, and renal stones may cause urinary symptoms but also produce other signs and symptoms that distinguish them from nonspecific urethritis.

328. The answer is A. *(Anderson, ed 9. pp 1860-1864.)* "Fibroids" of the uterus are among the most common abnormalities seen in uteri surgically removed in the United States in women of reproductive age. They arise in the myometrium, submucosally, subserosally, and midwall, both singly and several at a time. Sharply circumscribed, they are benign, smooth muscle tumors that are firm, gray-white, and whorled on cut section. Their malignant counterpart, leiomyosarcoma of the uterus, is quite rare in the de novo state and arises even more rarely from an antecedent leiomyoma. Whereas cell pleomorphism, tissue necrosis, and cytologic atypia per se are established criteria in assessing malignancy in tumors generally, they are important to the pathologist in uterine fibroids only if mitoses are also present. Regardless of cellularity or atypicality, if 10 or more mitoses are present in 10 separate high-power microscopic fields, the lesion is leiomyosarcoma. If 5 or fewer mitoses are present in 10 fields with bland morphology, the leiomyoma is going to behave in a benign fashion. Problems arise when the mitotic counts range between 3 and 7 per 10 fields with varying degrees of cell and tissue atypicality. These equivocal lesions should be regarded by both pathologist and clinician as "gray-area" smooth muscle tumors of unpredictable biologic behavior. Fortunately, the "gray-area" leiomyoma of the uterus is rarely seen. Thus mitoses are the most important criteria in assessing malignancy in smooth muscle tumors of the uterus.

329. The answer is E. *(Robbins, ed 4. pp 1100-1102.)* Of all the choices given, human papilloma virus (HPV) condyloma without dysplasia is the only lesion that can be histologically discriminated from the others. The typical HPV condyloma has hyperplastic squamous mucosa that shows progressive maturation from the stratum germinativum to the surface that is often parakeratotic, without cells of dysplasia or malignancy. There often are vacuolated squamous cells in several layers of the mucosa. However, condylomas, whether arising in the female or the male genital areas, may have atypia or dysplasia, or even be associated histologically with carcinoma. If present, these features must be commented upon in a pathology report. Condyloma not otherwise specified indicates that none of these disorders of growth are present along with it. Bowen's disease and erythroplasia of Queyrat are different clinical forms of squamous cell carcinoma in situ. Erythroplasia of Queyrat is a specialized form of squamous carcinoma in situ or severe dysplasia occurring on the glans penis mainly. It is characterized by a moist, macular, spreading red surface. It usually occurs in males of advanced age. Bowen's disease is also squamous carcinoma in situ but may have an association with malignancies of the viscera. Bowenoid papulosis refers to multiple, small, banal-appearing clinical papules on the vulvar or penile surfaces; it histologically shows features of Bowen's disease, and for all practical purposes cannot be distinguished from that disease on histologic grounds only. It is a rather new entity, histologically similar to carcinoma in situ, and it behaves as a self-healing and reversible lesion. Bowenoid papulosis usually occurs in young patients and is often associated with condylomas.

330. The answer is E. *(Robbins, ed 4. pp 1142-1144.)* Although the cervical intraepithelial neoplasia (CIN) system is not accepted by all workers in gynecology, many large centers are now using it for reporting cervical dysplasias. The system was created to circumvent and alleviate interpretation difficulties for pathologists, because cervical dysplasia includes a spectrum of diseases that, in many cases, eventuate in carcinoma in situ followed by a stage of microinvasion. The squamous mucosa is examined for atypical squamous cells and the thickness of the total mucosa occupied by them. CIN-1 represents less than one third thickness (mild dysplasia); CIN-2 represents one-third to two-thirds thickness (moderate dysplasia); CIN-3 represents two-thirds to the entire thickness occupied by abnormal cells (severe dysplasia, carcinoma in situ). It should be remembered that not all forms of cervical dysplasia inevitably go on to the next higher stage of disease, because some are reversible.

331. The answer is D. *(Robbins, ed 4. pp 1103-1104, 1108-1109.)* The condition illustrated is cryptorchidism, failure of the testis to descend into the scrotum. It is present in up to 1 percent of males after puberty. The testis is small, brown, and atrophic grossly. Microscopically, the tubules are atrophic with thickened basement membranes. The interstitial cells are usually prominent and occasional focal proliferations of Sertoli cells may be seen. The incidence of malignancy is increased by a factor of 30 to 50 and this risk is greater for abdominal than for inguinal location. Seminoma is the most common malignancy. The risk of malignancy is not reduced by orchiopexy. There is a smaller but definite risk of malignancy in the contralateral, correctly placed testis.

332. The answer is E. *(Anderson, ed 9. pp 856-857. Robbins, ed 4. pp 1089-1090.)* Malacoplakia is an uncommon chronic inflammatory disease of unknown cause, characterized by soft yellow mucosal plaques, infiltration of large histiocytes containing phagolysosomes, and intracytoplasmic and extracellular laminated calcospherules, Michaelis-Gutmann (MG) bodies. While malacoplakia usually involves the mucosa of the urinary bladder, it occurs also in extravesical sites such as the colon, lungs, kidneys, prostate, and brain. It occurs with greater frequency in the immunosuppressed. Histologically, the plaques contain numerous, large, foamy or granular macrophages that are PAS-positive and often include bacterial debris. Laminated, mineralized MG bodies are also numerous in, and between, macrophages. The cause of malacoplakia is not clear, but it has been associated with *E. coli* infections and is thought to be due to defective removal by macrophages of phagocytosed bacteria with overloaded phagosomes and MG bodies resulting from calcium deposition on the phagosomes. In recent reports, however, cerebral malacoplakia was not associated with bacterial infection.

333. The answer is D. *(Robbins, ed 4. pp 1153-1155.)* Endometrial adenocarcinoma appears to be increasing in frequency in the United States, especially in younger women. It is now accepted that a high estrogen-to-progestin ratio predisposes to the development of this tumor. At menopause, estrogen in the form of estrone continues to be produced in the adrenal glands, and the amounts are directly proportional to body fat. This continues in a milieu in which progesterone is at a minimum because of noncycling. These factors explain why obese women are at an increased risk during and after menopause. Diabetes and hypertension also are associated factors, but they are more likely to be effects of obesity than isolated risk factors for developing cancer. Endometrial adenocarcinoma is nearly always preceded by endometrial hyperplasia in some form. This, of course, is not documented in every case because not every patient has had a diagnostic dilatation and curettage of the endometrium prior to development of the carcinoma. Furthermore, endometrial hyperplasia does not always lead to adenocarcinoma.

334. The answer is D. *(Anderson, ed 9. pp 1688-1690.)* Benign cystic teratomas constitute about 10 percent of cystic ovarian tumors. The cysts contain greasy sebaceous material mixed with a variable amount of hair. The cysts' walls contain skin and skin appendages, including sebaceous glands and hair follicles. A variety of other tissues, such as cartilage, bone, tooth, thyroid, respiratory tract epithelium, and intestinal tissue, may be found. The presence of skin and skin appendages gives the tumor its other name, "dermoid" cyst. Dermoid cysts are benign, but in less than 2 percent, one element may become malignant, most frequently the squamous epithelium.

335. The answer is C. *(Robbins, ed 4. pp 1040-1041.)* Many diseases involve hematuria, and a few diseases occur in the setting of an upper respiratory infection or of upper respiratory signs and symptoms (streptococcal glomerulonephritis, Henoch-Schönlein purpura, Wegener's granulomatosis, and bacterial endocarditis with embolism), but when the hematuria follows within 1 to 1½ days of onset of an upper respiratory infection without skin lesions in a young patient, IgA nephropathy (Berger's disease) should be considered. This disease involves the deposition of IgA in the mesangium of the glomeruli. Light microscopic examination may suggest the disease, but renal biopsy immunofluorescence must be performed to confirm it. This disorder is not at all uncommon and may become recurrent, with proteinuria that may approach nephrotic syndrome proportions. Serum levels of IgA may be elevated. A small percentage of patients may progress to renal failure over a period of years.

336. The answer is C. *(Robbins, ed 4. p 1138.)* Adenocarcinomas of the vagina and cervix have existed for years, but have increased in young women whose mothers had received diethylstilbestrol (DES) while they had been pregnant. DES was used in the past to terminate an attack of threatened abortion and thereby stabilize the pregnancy. However, a side effect of this therapy proved to be a particular form of adenocarcinoma called clear cell carcinoma. This phenomenon was elucidated by Herpses and Scully in 1970. This unique adenocarcinoma was discovered in daughters between the ages of 15 and 20 of those women who had received DES. The tumor, which carries a poor prognosis, has at least three histologic patterns. One is a tubulopapillary configuration, followed by sheets of clear cells and glands lined by clear cells, and solid areas of relatively undifferentiated cells. Many of the cells have cytoplasm that protrudes into the lumen and produces a "hobnail" (nodular) appearance. Prior to the development of adenocarcinoma, a form of adenosis consisting of glands with clear cytoplasm that resembles that of the endocervix can be seen. This has been termed *vaginal adenosis* and may be a precursor of clear cell carcinoma. Clinically adenosis of the vagina is manifested by red, moist granules superimposed on the pink-white vaginal mucosa.

337. The answer is A. *(Robbins, ed 4. pp 1158-1164.)* Malignant tumors of the ovary most commonly occur between the ages of 40 and 64. These, in the main, arise from the surface epithelium, which takes its origin from cells of the müllerian system. These cells are also referred to as *surface* or *coelomic epithelium.* The müllerian system has the ability to form lining cells of the fallopian tubes, endometrium, and endocervical gland epithelium. Hence, many malignant tumors that take their origin from the surface coelomic epithelium of the ovary resemble these structures. Examples include the borderline serous tumor, serous cystadenocarcinoma, serous cystadenofibrocarcinoma, borderline mucinous tumor, mucinous cystadenocarcinoma, endometrioid carcinoma, undifferentiated carcinoma, malignant Brenner tumor, and clear cell adenocarcinoma. Stem cells from the urogenital ridge can give rise to any genitourinary structure. Hilar cells represent small clusters and cords of androgen-producing cells. These presumably give rise to sex cord and Sertoli-Leydig cell tumors. Stromal cell tumors include granulosa cell tumors, theca cell tumors, thecomas, and fibromas. Germ cell tumors give rise to malignant and benign teratomas, including the cystic form (dermoid cyst), dysgerminoma, endodermal sinus tumor, choriocarcinoma, and mixed germ cell tumors.

338. The answer is C. *(Robbins, ed 4. pp 1158-1163.)* Ovarian cystadenomas are common neoplasms that are bilateral in 15 to 40 percent of patients and are frequently papillary. The less malignant lesions tend to be more papillary. Ovarian cystadenomas originate in surface epithelial cells from the müllerian system. The papillae may show complex arborization with an increase in cell layers without stromal invasion; in such cases, the tumors are classified as borderline malignant because of their less aggressive clinical course. Unlike true cystadenocarcinomas, the presence of peritoneal dissemination in cystadenomas of borderline malignancy does not appear to influence the clinical course.

339. The answer is A. *(Robbins, ed 4. p 1170.)* The eponym "Krukenberg's tumor" designates a bilateral ovarian neoplasm that is almost always metastatic from cancer of the gastrointestinal tract, particularly the stomach. This type of tumor is characterized microscopically by a diffuse infiltration of signet-ring cells containing abundant mucin and by areas of mucoid degeneration. Krukenberg's tumor designates a metastatic carcinoma to the ovary that is, at cursory examination, deceptively bland.

340. The answer is B. *(Anderson, ed 9. pp 882-886.)* Most malignant germ cell tumors of the gonads, specifically the testis, typically occur in the younger male between the ages of 22 and 35. The seminoma has several types, most of which are found also within the younger ages. The classic seminoma is populated by differentiated seminiferous tubule-type epithelium with intervening lymphocytes, while the anaplastic seminoma contains an increase in mitoses and a moderate degree of anaplasia. The spermatocytic seminoma, however, occurs in older patients, often between 55 and 65, and is a soft, yellowish, sometimes mucoid tumor that microscopically has several cell types: classic intermediate-sized germ cells, smaller secondary spermatocytic-type cells, and large mononuclear and multinuclear giant cells. Polyembryoma and embryonal carcinoma are related, occur in the younger patient, and are less common than the seminomas. The most malignant germ cell tumor of the testis is the choriocarcinoma, which is characterized by large cytotrophoblastic and syncytiotrophoblastic cells. Teratocarcinomas are tumors of more than one histologic type that may contain seminomatous or embryonal components, or both.

341. The answer is E. *(Robbins, ed 4. pp 1160–1163.)* Primary ovarian tumors have a rather high degree of bilateral involvement compared with tumors of other bilateral organs. Bilaterality could reflect either concurrent simultaneous primary tumors or vascular and lymphatic spread from one side to the other. The ovarian tumor with the highest rate of bilaterality (70 percent) is the serous cystadenocarcinoma. Serous cystadenomas have a 30 percent rate of bilaterality, while mucinous cystadenomas are bilateral in about 5 percent of cases. In contrast, mucinous cystadenocarcinomas are bilateral in 20 percent of cases, and endometrioid carcinoma is higher at about 45 percent. There is a higher probability of extension of endometrioid carcinoma outside of the ovaries when it presents with bilaterality.

342. The answer is D. *(Anderson, ed 9. p 891.)* The adenomatoid tumor is benign and is the most common tumor of the epididymis. Its origin is probably the mesothelium. It presents as a small, firm, gray-white nodule less than 5 cm in diameter; similar tumors occur in the fallopian tube, ovary, and posterior uterus. Histology reveals gland-like, mesothelium-lined spaced and fibrous connective tissue stroma with smooth muscle fibers. Androblastoma, or Sertoli cell tumor, is a sex cord testicular tumor, often benign; tuberculous epididymitis presents multiple confluent tubercles with caseation. Carcinomas of epididymis and adjacent structures occur, but are very rare. Adrenocortical rests are common, but usually too small for clinical detection.

343. The answer is C. *(Anderson, ed 9. pp 300, 324, 1645. Tam, N Engl J Med 310:1146, 1984.)* At least 50 percent of the infections of the uterine cervix in women in the United States today are caused by *Chlamydia trachomatis,* which is an intracellular obligate bacterium that can be identified by direct immunofluorescence using monoclonal antibodies. In addition to venereal transmission, *Chlamydia* also may cause psittacosis, trachoma, and neonatal infections. *Campylobacter* causes intestinal infections with diarrheal syndromes, while *Calymmatobacterium* causes granuloma inguinale, a venereally transmitted disease consisting of painful ulcers, which histologically shows granulomas with coccobacillary microorganisms within macrophages. The organism is antigenically related to *Klebsiella*. The gonococcus of the *Neisseria* genus causes gonorrhea but is less common than *Chlamydia*.

344. The answer is C. *(Koss, ed 3. pp 182-190.)* Predominance of parabasal squamous cells in a lateral vaginal wall smear indicates low estrogen effect and atrophic epithelium, as in atrophic postmenopausal mucosa. A similar picture is seen with the relatively atrophic mucosa of prepuberty, lactation, or primary amenorrhea. Specimens for hormone evaluation should be obtained from the lateral vaginal wall and hormone assessment should not be made without knowing the patient's age, menstrual history, and whether she received exogenous hormones. Predominance of flat, superficial squamous cells with pyknotic nuclei indicates unopposed estrogen effect (ovulation or midcycle). Predominance of intermediate squamous cells is seen most often in the late luteal or secretory phase and in pregnancy.

345. The answer is B. *(Robbins, ed 4. pp 1090-1094.)* Approximately 90 percent of carcinomas of the bladder are of transitional cell type. They are more common in men. Known etiological factors include cigarette smoking, persistent mucosal inflammation, exposure to certain chemicals, notably beta-naphthylamine, and administration of the immunosuppressive agent cyclophosphamide (Cytoxan). Infection by *Schistosoma haematobium* is associated with squamous cell cancer. All transitional cell cancers, regardless of grade, tend to recur; the frequency of recurrence increases with the tumor grade.

346. The answer is E (all). *(Anderson, ed 9. p 815.)* The photomicrograph shows focal glomerulonephritis with crescent formation and focal hypercellularity involving only one portion of the glomerulus. Focal glomerulonephritis involves some glomeruli, but not all, and may involve the entire glomerulus (global) or only parts of the glomerulus (segmental). The photomicrograph demonstrates focal segmental glomerulonephritis, which may be seen in systemic diseases as well as disorders affecting only the kidney. Hypercellularity involved several mesangia with proliferation of epithelial cells lining Bowman's capsule near the damaged capillary loops. This process is referred to as *crescent formation.* The disease may be seen in bacterial endocarditis and other systemic infections. Immunologic disorders causing focal segmental glomerulonephritis may include IgA focal glomerulonephritis, systemic lupus erythematosus, polyarteritis nodosa, and Schönlein-Henoch purpura (anaphylactoid purpura). IgA focal glomerulonephritis, also known as Berger's disease, has deposits of IgA and some IgG in the involved mesangium as demonstrated by immunofluorescence. Alport's syndrome is a hereditary form of chronic renal disease that may be associated with neural deafness and death at an early age, usually less than 30. Large collections of foam cells are also seen in the renal cortex in these patients. Electron microscopy shows splitting of the glomerular basements accompanied by small, electron-dense granules.

347. The answer is B (1, 3). *(Robbins, ed 4. pp 1029-1031.)* Acute poststreptococcal glomerulonephritis usually affects children 5 to 30 days after a streptococcal infection. It is associated with decreased serum complement and increased ASO titer. Immune complexes seen as electron-dense deposits are bound within the glomerular basement membrane on the epithelial side. Ninety-five percent of affected patients recover without sequelae.

348. The answer is A (1, 2, 3). *(Robbins, ed 4. pp 1044-1047.)* Diabetes is a major cause of renal disease. It affects the glomeruli with resultant glomerulosclerosis, fibrin caps, and capsular drops. It also affects the renal vasculature, where it causes atheroma of the major renal arteries and hyaline arteriolosclerosis of both afferent and efferent arterioles. Acute infection of the renal pyramids occurs and in combination with impaired circulation to the papillae may lead to papillary necrosis. The finding at autopsy of acute pyelonephritis is increased in the diabetic, but this is thought to be due to the terminal event, and it is not firmly established that acute pyelonephritis is increased in the living diabetic population.

349. The answer is D (4). *(Robbins, ed 4. pp 1069, 1070.)* The group of renal diseases associated with microangiopathic hemolytic anemia includes both childhood and adult hemolytic-uremic syndrome (HUS), thrombotic thrombocytopenic purpura, and scleroderma. Endothelial injury and intravascular coagulation occur in all. HUS is characterized by acute renal failure, microangiopathic hemolytic anemia, and thrombocytopenia and is one of the main causes of acute renal failure in children. Prodromal features in children include a gastrointestinal or respiratory tract infection. Lupus erythematosus does not occur in very young children. Acute poststreptococcal glomerulonephritis occurs in older children, is a proliferative lesion, and is not usually associated with hemolytic anemia or fibrin deposition. Lipoid nephrosis shows no glomerular changes with light microscopy.

350. The answer is A (1, 2, 3). *(Anderson, ed 9. pp 826, 827. Robbins, ed 4. pp 1069, 1070.)* Endothelial injury is considered to be an initiating pathologic event, especially in HUS associated with gram-negative infections, predominantly infection with verocytotoxin-producing *E. coli*. The verocytotoxins of *E. coli*, which infects up to 75 percent of the patients, are cytotoxic to endothelium. Hypertension exists in about 50 percent of the patients, but the relative lack of CNS involvement helps to distinguish HUS from thrombotic thrombocytopenic purpura in which there is usually more general involvement with thrombi formed in several organs.

351. The answer is B (1, 3). *(Anderson, ed 9. pp 847-849.)* The neoplasms of renal cell carcinoma are produced as spheres that have diameters ranging from 3 to

15 cm and have been described as tissues that are bright or golden yellow, gray, tan in areas of low lipid content, white in areas of fibrosis and coagulative necrosis, or any combination of these colors. Renal cell carcinomas commonly arise from the upper pole, characteristically invade the renal veins, and then may metastasize unpredictably, slowly, or explosively to the lungs, bone, brain, regional lymph nodes, liver, adrenals, eye (sometimes), and vagina, or any one of these. The metastases often proceed asymptomatically and, when detected, may be diagnosed as a tumor of the lung or some other affected organ or tissue instead of as primary renal cell carcinoma. In the "solid cell" type of tumor, cytological detail persists and cells are cuboid; in the "clear cell" type, although cytoplasm is completely vacuolated, cell membranes remain intact.

352. The answer is E (all). *(Robbins, ed 4. pp 1044-1047.)* Thickening of the capillary basement membrane is a universal finding in diabetic kidney disease and consists of diffuse thickening as is seen in vasculopathy in other organ sites in diabetes. This has to be verified by ultrastructural examination by EM. Additionally, the mesangium widens and tubular basement membranes also thicken in diabetes. Thickening is produced by hyaline-like material, which reacts with the PAS stain. This may result from glycosylation of the proteins of the basement membrane. Thickening is probably also contributed by an increase in collagen type 4, as well as in the basement membrane glycoprotein laminen; however, the polyanionic proteoglycans are decreased. This may contribute to the increased permeability and consequent leakage of cationic proteins into the urine. Diffuse glomerulosclerosis results from an increase in the mesangial matrix as well as an increase in mesangial cells. This increase in matrix will also react with the PAS stain. Eventually, with continuing disease the glomerular tufts will become obliterated and yield a sclerosed, acidophilic tuft. At this stage the afferent and probably efferent arterioles will also be thickened and appear hyalinized.

Nodular glomerulosclerosis (Kimmelstiel-Wilson disease, intercapillary glomerulosclerosis) appears as laminated hyaline nodules at the peripheries of the glomerulus covered by what appears to be patent capillary loops. They may resemble amyloid and if they are present, amyloid stain should be done. Not always present, but highly characteristic of diabetic glomerulopathy are fibrin caps and capsular drops. The fibrin cap is a deposit that overlies a peripheral capillary within the glomerulus and consists of acidophilic deposits between the basement membrane and the endothelial cells. Capsular drops are PAS-positive proteinaceous foci that compose a thickening of the parietal layer of Bowman's capsule, giving the appearance of being free within the urinary ultrafiltrate.

353. The answer is A (1, 2, 3). *(Robbins, ed 4. pp 1033-1041.)* While many varieties of glomerulonephritis can produce the nephrotic syndrome, a few disorders will virtually always produce it. Included in the latter group are focal (segmental) glomerulosclerosis, membranous glomerulonephritis (GN), lipoid nephrosis, membranoproliferative glomerulonephritis, systemic diseases (such as amyloidosis and systemic lupus erythematosus), some tumors, hepatitis B, syphilis, drugs such as penicillamine, and certain allergies. Light microscopy shows very little change in glomeruli in lipoid nephrosis, and a diffuse absence of glomerular epithelial foot processes is noted with electron microscopy. Membranoproliferative GN is characterized by an increase in mesangial cellularity accompanied by splitting of the glomerular basement membranes ("double contour"). Membranous GN shows electron-dense deposits of immunoglobulin in the subepithelial portion of the basement membrane. The nephrotic syndrome includes massive albuminuria with significant loss of protein (more than 3 to 5 g of protein) in 24 hours, consequent reduced plasma albumin (less than 3 g/dl), hyperlipidemia, and anasarca (generalized edema).

354. The answer is E (all). *(Robbins, ed 4. pp 1062-1069.)* Many pathologic processes affecting the kidney can lead to hypertension. The three main categories are renovascular, renal parenchymal, and urinary tract obstruction. The renin-angiotensin system has been implicated in renovascular hypertension but has not been proved to be of etiologic importance in the other two categories. The most common parenchymal diseases leading to hypertension are pyelonephritis and hydronephrosis.

355. The answer is D (4). *(Robbins, ed 4. pp 1043-1047.)* Ultrastructural studies reveal dense deposits in the mesangium of the glomerulus in addition to deposition of IgG, IgA, IgM, and complement (C_3), as seen by immunofluorescence microscopy. With light microscopy, fibrin and platelets also appear to be present. IgA is the immunoglobulin most commonly found in anaphylactoid purpura glomerulonephritis and may be associated with elevated serum levels of IgA.

356. The answer is E (all). *(Richart, Cancer 60:1951-1959, 1987. Robbins, ed 4. p 1142.)* Cervical squamous cell cancer and its precursors (dysplasia) are considered to be sexually transmitted diseases. Women having sexual intercourse at an early age or with multiple male partners, particularly those with penile condylomas, are at high risk for development of genital tract squamous neoplasms. Herpes simplex virus (HSV) type 2 was considered an important cause, but is now thought to have a role only in conjunction with human papilloma virus (HPV) types 16/18. Existence of the genome of HPV types 6, 11, 16, 18, 31, and 33 has been documented by DNA hybridization methods in several genital lesions including condylomas, cervical intraepithelial neoplasia (CIN) carcinoma in situ, and invasive cervical cancer. In most studies HPV 6 and 11 were confined to lesions with a good prognosis such as condylomas and mild dysplasia (CIN I), whereas HPV 16 and 18 were found predominantly in CIN III (severe dysplasia and carcinoma in situ) and in invasive carcinoma.

357. The answer is A (1, 2, 3). *(Braunwald, ed 11. p 1582. Robbins, ed 4. pp 1121-1125.)* Over 95 percent of prostatic cancers are adenocarcinomas. In nearly 75 percent of cases adenocarcinoma of the prostate arises in the posterior lobe, usually in a subcapsular location. The lateral lobes are the next, much less frequent site. Nodular hyperplasia occurs in the periurethral region. When prostatic cancer is extracapsular or metastatic (commonly osteoblastic metastases to pelvis and lumbar vertebrae), serum tumor markers such as prostatic acid phosphatase (PAP) are detectable by standard assays. Tumor growth may be inhibited by estrogen therapy; it is not estrogen-dependent. Invasion of capsule, blood vessels, and perineural spaces is useful in diagnosis of well-differentiated tumor. Diagnosis may include needle biopsy or fine needle aspiration (80 percent accuracy).

358. The answer is E (all). *(Robbins, ed 4. p 1095.)* Obstruction of the bladder neck from any cause will lead to urinary retention within the bladder with consequent dilatation and an inability to empty the bladder completely on micturition. The patient may complain of having marked nocturnal frequency owing to a combination of a sense of urgency caused by being in the recumbent position with a "full" bladder and the inability to empty the bladder completely because of the obstruction. This leads to urinary stasis, which provides a potential culture medium for bacteria, especially such gram-negative coliform bacilli as *Proteus, Klebsiella,* and *Escherichia.* There is a potential hazard of developing gram-negative septicemia from this focus. The chronic retention and dilatation lead to hypertrophy of the bladder muscle with trabeculation of the submucosa and mucosa. Causes are usually prostatic in the male (benign prostatic nodular hyperplasia or carcinoma) and extrinsic pressure in the woman exerted by masses in the cervix or rectum. Early surgery is imperative.

359. The answer is B (1, 3). *(Robbins, ed 4. pp 1171-1172.)* Ectopic pregnancy is a potentially life-threatening condition if it is not treated by removal before rupture and hemorrhage with fatal exsanguination. The most common location for extrauterine implantation is the fallopian tube (more than 85 percent of cases), with rare implantation in the ovary or abdomen. If the tubal implantation has existed from 1 to 4 weeks, the beta-HcG test result is likely to be negative; thus a negative result does *not* exclude pregnancy. It is always worthwhile to repeat a laboratory test when the result is unexpected. Tubal pregnancy is not uncommon and should always be considered if endometrial curettings suggest gestational change without chorionic villi.

360. The answer is C (2, 4). *(Anderson, ed 9. pp 808, 818-819.)* There are numerous causes of nephrotic syndrome (NS), including immune complex diseases, diabetes, amyloidosis, toxemia of pregnancy, and such circulating disturbances as bilateral renal vein thrombosis, but NS occurring in small children (under 3 years of age) should suggest the possibility of the renal disease known as minimal change nephropathy, which is synonymous with "foot process" disease or nil disease. This peculiar entity presents clinically as insidious nephrotic syndrome, characteristically occurring in younger children, but also seen in adults (rarely), with hypoalbuminemia, edema, hyperlipidemia, massive proteinuria, and lipiduria. The glomeruli are known for their rather normal appearance on light microscopy—at worst, there is mild and focal sclerosis. Electron microscopy is necessary for demonstrating characteristic attenuation and flattening of the foot processes of the podocytes attached to the Bowman's space side of the glomerular basement membrane. The podocytes may revert to normal (with steroid immunosuppressive therapy), or the foot-process attenuation may persist to some extent, in which case the proteinuria also persists. To date, no immune complex deposits or abnormalities of the glomerular basement membrane or mesangium have been demonstrated ultrastructurally.

361. The answer is B (1, 3). *(Anderson, ed 9. pp 1667-1668.)* Neisseria gonorrhoeae is a very common bacterium that causes acute pelvic inflammatory disease with salpingitis in this country as a result of venereal infection. Tuboovarian abscesses may develop from this bacterium, as well as other bacteria, but these organisms are susceptible to penicillin therapy. In the presence of unresponsiveness to penicillin, consideration should be given to *Bacteroides* species, which are important anaerobic gram-negative bacilli and are generally refractory to penicillin. These anaerobic bacteria may produce serious infections if uncontrolled. Chlamydiae, while considered to be nongonococcal in origin, are nevertheless important agents in venereal transmission and often are contracted at the same time that *Neisseria* species are. When the gonococcus is adequately treated with penicillin, and symptoms continue, there may have been concurrent infection with chlamydia that is not responsive to penicillin but is sensitive to tetracycline. Adenoviruses are responsible for keratoconjunctivitis, tracheobronchitis, pneumonia in children, acute gastroenteritis, and occasionally hemorrhagic cystitis, but are not ordinarily causative in pelvic inflammatory disease.

362. The answer is A (1, 2, 3). *(Robbins, ed 4. pp 1150-1151.)* Cystic endometrial hyperplasia refers to the abnormal growth of endometrium associated with either an absolute or a relative estrogen excess. These are common findings at the time of menopause and in conditions causing an absolute excess of estrogen—e.g., Stein-Leventhal syndrome, functioning granulosa and thecal cell ovarian tumors, and the exogenous administration of estrogenic substances. The microscopic findings in an endometrial biopsy are dominated by the marked dilatation of the endometrial glands, giving the tissue section the appearance of Swiss cheese. The glands are lined by benign columnar epithelium that is nonsecretory.

363. The answer is A (1, 2, 3). *(Gottlieb, Ann Intern Med 99:208, 1983. Reichert, Am J Pathol 112:357, 1983.)* The most common tumor being seen in homosexual men with acquired immunodeficiency syndrome is Kaposi's sarcoma either locally in the skin or disseminated. Other tumors in this population being seen with increasing frequency are lymphomas, including those in the central nervous system, and solid tumors of the oral and anal regions. The latter have included squamous cell carcinomas, especially of the oropharynx but also of the perianal skin. The cloacogenic carcinoma of the anorectal region is a deep tumor arising in the junction of the squamocolumnar mucosa; it may have a poor prognosis if composed predominantly of undifferentiated small cells.

364. The answer is D (4). *(Robbins, ed 4. pp 1012-1018.)* The unique structure and composition of the glomerular basement membrane and associated cells account for the formation of the plasma ultrafiltrate referred to as *urine*. The glomerular basement membrane is approximately 320 nm wide in the normal human with a central electron-dense lamina densa and electron-lucent lamina rara interna and externa with fenestrated endothelial cells immediately adjacent to the capillaries and the visceral epithelial cells (podocytes). Glomerular basement membrane is made up of collagen type 4, with laminen especially concentrated on both laminae rarae. Clustered also on both laminae rarae are polyanionic proteoglycans (especially heparan sulfate), which are thought to play a major role in the exclusion of albumin in the urinary filtrate by a mechanism of charge dependence restriction. This is based on the electronegative charge of the proteoglycans and the anionic charges of albumin. The mechanism is based on different isoelectric points. Thus it is felt that the glomerulus, because of these proteoglycans, may be able to discriminate materials passing through the glomerulus according to electronegative charge. Glomerular basement membrane does function by exclusion of materials based on size. Mesangial cells, by nature of their contractility, are thought to control intraglomerular blood flow under neurohormonal stimulation. Mesangial cells are not thought to function in filtration per se. The parietal cells lining the Bowman's membrane may function as a barrier but do not participate in the ultrafiltration. The fenestrated endothelial cells and podocytes are part of the filtering membrane but probably play a minor role compared with the glomerular polyanion barrier.

365. The answer is D (4). *(Robbins, ed 4. pp 1012-1014.)* It has been recently shown that polyanionic molecules at sites on the luminal endothelial cells retard anions by electronegativity forces, aiding the transport of cationic proteins. They may greatly increase vascular permeability, especially in the renal glomerulus. The glomerular basement membrane contains the glycoprotein entactin, fibronectin, collagen type IV, laminen, and polyanionic proteoglycans (heparan sulfate) found at sites on both laminae rarae. The glomerular filtration barrier is made possible by these polyanions. The podocyte is attached to the lamina rara externa on the epithelial (urine filtrate) side of the glomerular basement membrane. Desmin is an intermediate filament protein found in fibroblasts and muscle cells. Bowman's capsule epithelial cells line the inner side of the glomerulus and are bathed in urinary ultrafiltrate. Fibronectin, a connective tissue protein formed by endothelial cells, fibroblasts, and macrophages, stabilizes endothelial cell attachments and functions in wound healing.

366. The answer is A (1, 2, 3). *(Robbins, ed 4. pp 1152-1153.)* The condition illustrated is a uterine leiomyoma (fibroid). This is an extremely common tumor occurring in up to 25 percent of women of reproductive age. The cause is unknown, but the growth is estrogen-dependent and for this reason the tumor may enlarge rapidly during pregnancy. If the tumor becomes very large, areas within it may undergo softening followed by liquefaction and cystic degeneration. Fibroids tend to regress in the postmenopausal period; with atrophy they become collagenous and calcification often occurs.

367. The answer is E (all). *(Robbins, ed 4. pp 1167-1168.)* The signs of hyperestrogenism produced by ovarian neoplasms, such as the granulosa cell tumor or a thecoma, are most obvious clinically as precocious puberty in a child or menstrual abnormalities and endometrial hyperplasia in a postmenopausal woman. These tumors may produce uterine enlargement as a result of muscle hypertrophy and marked endometrial hyperplasia.

368. The answer is D (4). *(Robbins, ed 4. pp 1168-1169.)* Meigs' syndrome is a benign ovarian fibroma associated with ascites and occasionally with pleural effusion, usually right-sided. After the fibroma is removed, the ascites and pleural effusion will normally disappear. Since the pleural space does not contain neoplastic cells in Meigs' syndrome, intrapleural administration of chemotherapeutic agents is not required therapy.

369. The answer is D (4). *(Graves, N Engl J Med 312:338, 1985.)* Measuring acid phosphatase intracellularly by the immunohistochemical method for in situ cells as in a needle biopsy is specific for prostate source, as is the same determination for prostatic specific antigen. Circulating plasma levels of prostatic acid phosphatase are elevated in circumstances of metastatic prostate adenocarcinoma. Alkaline phosphatases are found within the liver, placenta, and bone. Measurement of a recently described protein in semen is highly specific for seminal fluid, and the detection of the presence of p30 antigen in vaginal fluid is conclusive evidence that coitus has taken place. The test is an ELISA determination.

370. The answer is D (4). *(Robbins, ed 4. pp 1105-1106.)* Mumps orchitis rarely occurs before puberty. Testicular involvement, most often unilateral, commonly begins between the fifth and tenth days of illness during subsidence of parotid swelling. Some degree of atrophy, caused by pressure necrosis, occurs in about one-third to one-half of the cases of orchitis. The involvement of the testis is usually spotty, however, and seldom results in sterility.

371. The answer is E (all). *(Anderson, ed 9. pp 379-382.)* Cytomegalic inclusion disease is diagnosed in the immunosuppressed or AIDS patient by finding large intranuclear inclusions surrounded by a clear halo in enlarged cells in urinary sediment, in sputum or bronchial lavage, in spinal fluid specimens, or in liver biopsy. Small intracytoplasmic inclusions may be found. Cytomegalovirus (CMV) is a DNA member of the herpesvirus group that causes disseminated disease, including interstitial pneumonitis in the debilitated or immunosuppressed adult. Disseminated infection with CMV in AIDS is associated with pneumonitis, hepatitis, idiopathic ulcerative colitis, encephalitis, and retinitis. Rising antibody titers may not be detectable for up to 4 weeks after primary infection and early diagnosis may be achieved by finding typical inclusion bodies in cytologic or biopsy specimens.

372. The answer is A (1, 2, 3). *(Robbins, ed 4. p 1138.)* Neoplasms of the vagina are rare, but of these squamous cell carcinoma is the most common. Vaginal clear cell adenocarcinoma occurs occasionally (1 or less per 1000) in girls in their late teens whose mothers had received diethylstilbestrol during pregnancy. In about one-third of cases such cancers arise in the cervix. More frequently, in about half of the population at risk, small glandular or microcystic lesions appear in the mucosa— vaginal adenosis. These benign lesions appear as red, velvety foci and are lined by mucus-secreting or ciliated columnar cells. From these areas the rarer clear cell adenocarcinoma arises. Sarcoma botryoides, producing soft polypoid grape-like masses, is another rare primary vaginal cancer found usually in infants and children under age 5. It is a rhabdomyosarcoma that can also occur in the urinary bladder.

373. The answer is C (2, 4). *(Robbins, ed 4. pp 1104-1105.)* The condition illustrated is acute orchitis. There is hemorrhage and inflammation in and between tubules with disruption of spermatogenesis. Bacteria are present in the tubules. Orchitis is somewhat less common than epididymitis and, when present, is usually due to extension of infection from the urinary tract via epididymal lymphatics or the vas deferens. Infection is rarely blood-borne. *E. coli* and *C. trachomatis* are the most common pathogens. Sequelae include tubular atrophy and excretory duct obstruction, both of which may cause sterility. Chronic infection may occur. Interstitial cells are more likely to survive or regenerate, so sexual function is often retained.

374-376. The answers are: 374-B, 375-C, 376-E. *(Robbins, ed 4. pp 1031-1044.)* Membranoproliferative glomerulonephritis occurs in two types. Type I, which is associated with nephrotic syndrome, is driven by immune complexes; type II is associated with hematuria and chronic renal failure and in addition to immune complexes involves alternate complement activation. In either type there is mesangial proliferation accompanied by thickening of the glomerular basement membranes, and a special finding that often supports the diagnosis of membranoproliferative glomerulonephritis is the presence of actual splitting of the glomerular basement membranes. In type I there are subendothelial deposits of IgG, C3, C1, and C4. In type II there are dense deposits of C3 (dense-deposit disease) with or without IgG and no C1.

Membranous glomerulonephritis, on the other hand, rather than being driven by an immune complex is antibody-mediated and results in diffuse thickening of glomerular capillary walls by subepithelial deposits of IgG and C3 in a diffuse involvement of the glomeruli. These deposits are seen by fluorescence as granular deposits. Membranous glomerulonephritis is also associated with the nephrotic syndrome.

Goodpasture's syndrome is an acute serious disease often heralded by pulmonary hemorrhages and remarkable hemoptysis accompanied by acute glomerulonephritis that often is of the rapidly progressive form. Antiglomerular basement membrane antibodies are seen in Goodpasture's syndrome, which result in IgG linear deposits along the glomerular basement membranes. Also seen are marked and dramatic formations of epithelial cell crescents accompanied by infiltrates of monocytes and neutrophils with fibrin deposition and necrosis of epithelial and endothelial cells. There is no accompanying fragmentation of glomerular basement membranes as there is in membranoproliferative glomerulonephritis.

Glomerular hypercellularity with ingress of neutrophils characterizes poststreptococcal glomerulonephritis, while hyalinized ("dropped-out") glomeruli may be seen in any terminal glomerulonephritis but are best seen in the conditions of chronic renal failure caused by chronic glomerulonephritis.

377-379. The answers are: 377-A, 378-E, 379-E. *(Robbins, ed 4. pp 1044-1047, 1054-1055, 1059, 1066-1068.)* Renal arteriolar changes in malignant hypertension include fibrinoid necrosis of arterioles and hyperplastic arteriolonephrosis. Hyperplastic arteriolonephrosis is recognized by a proliferation of smooth muscle cells and fibrocytes and lamination of fibrinoid material with the blood vessel wall, which produces a concentric and laminated appearance. This condition differs from the lesion of hyaline nephrosclerosis, in which the arterioles demonstrate hyaline thickening only, without a proliferative cell component. The clinical course of malignant hypertension reflects the necrotizing and proliferative nature of the renal arteriolar changes in the disease, which can occur in a spectrum of underlying conditions, such as nephrosclerosis, pyelonephritis, glomerulonephritis, and progressive systemic sclerosis.

Diabetic (intercapillary) glomerulosclerosis (DG), or Kimmelstiel-Wilson disease, yields a characteristic mesangial matrix increase with peripheral, glomerular-tuft, sclerotic, round nodules. There is usually no mesangial cell increase, as is seen in the membranoproliferative glomerulopathies. DG may resemble amyloid glomerulopathy, however, and in doubtful cases the PAS-positive nodules of DG should not produce green birefringence under polarization after staining with Congo red. Other forms of diabetic nephropathy are hyaline arteriosclerosis, pyelonephritis, and necrotizing papillitis—a variant of pyelonephritis.

380-384. The answers are: 380-D, 381-A, 382-B, 383-A, 384-C. *(Robbins, ed 4. pp 1174-1178.)* The trophoblastic tumors include the benign hydatidiform mole, the invasive mole (chorioadenoma destruens), and choriocarcinoma. Hydatidiform mole occurs in the U.S. in about 1 in 2000 pregnancies. Both hydatidiform mole and choriocarcinoma produce high levels of human chorionic gonadotropin (HCG); the levels are extremely high in choriocarcinoma unless considerable tumor necrosis is present. Alpha-fetoprotein is not produced by trophoblastic tumors, in contrast to embryonal carcinoma and teratomas, which both may produce alpha-fetoprotein and human chorionic gonadotropin simultaneously. Choriocarcinoma shows the following incidence: 50 percent arise in moles, 25 percent follow abortion, and about 22 percent arise in normal pregnancy; the remainder originate in ectopic pregnancies and extragenital and genital teratomas, including teratoma of the testis. The cure rate for choriocarcinoma is very high (up to 80 percent) with chemotherapy of methotrexate and actinomycin.

385-388. The answers are: 385-C, 386-B, 387-A, 388-B. *(Robbins, ed 4. pp 1036-1038.)* Minimal change disease (MCD), or lipoid nephrosis, is the most common cause of the nephrotic syndrome in children (65 percent of cases; 10 to 20 percent of adult cases). In MCD loss or flattening of foot processes of epithelial cells occurs, but immunofluorescence shows no immunoglobulin or complement deposits. Renal biopsy may be required to differentiate early MCD from early membranous glomerulonephritis (MGN), but subepithelial immunoglobulin deposits are found in MGN and developed cases show diffuse thickening of the glomerular capillary wall. Glomeruli in MCD appear virtually normal by light microscopy. Rapid response to steroid therapy and excellent long-term prognosis characterize MCD.

Focal segmental glomerulosclerosis (FSG) accounts for about 10 to 15 percent of cases of nephrotic syndrome in both children and adults. The characteristic change in some glomeruli (focal) consists of areas of mesangial sclerosis with collapse of capillary loops spreading out from the central tufts. Other changes may include occlusion of capillary lumina by hyaline protein deposits (hyalinosis). Immunofluorescence shows IgM and C3, mostly in sclerotic mesangial areas. The electron-microscopic changes are mesangial sclerosis in affected glomeruli and fusion of foot processes in all glomeruli—changes similar to those seen in MCD. Most cases of FSG are idiopathic, but the nephrotic syndrome and FSG are found in more than 10 percent of patients with AIDS, as well as in chronic intravenous heroin users. Since T-cell function in AIDS is so abnormal, release of a toxic lymphokine could be responsible for the glomerular injury. Response to steroid therapy is poor and more than 50 percent of the patients die, or have persistent disease, within 10 years of diagnosis.

Nervous System

DIRECTIONS: Each question below contains five suggested responses. Select the **one best** response to each question.

389. Which of the following conditions is the most frequent cause of intracerebral hemorrhage?

(A) Ruptured aneurysm
(B) Trauma
(C) Blood dyscrasias
(D) Angiomas
(E) Hypertensive vascular disease

390. A 9-year-old boy who had been suffering from a gait disturbance for several weeks was found to have a posterior fossa mass on CT scan. The most likely cause for these findings is

(A) a berry aneurysm
(B) astrocytoma
(C) medulloblastoma
(D) oligodendroglioma
(E) pseudotumor cerebri

391. Tuberculous leptomeningitis is

(A) associated with smooth-walled cavities in the brain
(B) often associated with subdural effusion
(C) often a result of vertebral infection
(D) usually located over the cerebral convexities
(E) often part of miliary infection in children

392. A 55-year-old woman is suspected of having a brain tumor because of the onset of seizure activity. Computerized tomograms (CT scans) and skull x-rays demonstrate a mass in the right cerebral hemisphere that is markedly calcific. A high index of suspicion should exist for

(A) oligodendroglioma
(B) astrocytoma
(C) cerebral lymphoma
(D) metastatic carcinoma
(E) brown tumor

393. Retinoblastoma, the most common intraocular tumor of children, is associated with all the following EXCEPT

(A) occurrence in both familial and sporadic patterns
(B) unilateral and unifocal sporadic tumors
(C) inactivation of cancer suppressor genes
(D) poor prognosis even with treatment
(E) frequent histologic occurrence of rosettes

394. Which of the following cell populations of the central nervous system is the most rapidly affected by ischemia?

(A) Axis cylinders
(B) Neuronal nerve cell bodies
(C) Astrocytes
(D) Microglia
(E) Oligodendroglia

395. All the following have been commonly associated with pyogenic brain abscesses EXCEPT

(A) congenital heart disease
(B) sinusitis
(C) lung abscess
(D) liver abscess
(E) mastoiditis

396. Subdural hematomas occur most frequently in the

(A) supracerebellar region
(B) infracerebellar region
(C) cerebellopontine angle
(D) pituitary region
(E) cerebral hemisphere convexities

397. Select the disorder below that has the most clinicopathologic features in common with postvaccinal encephalomyelitis.

(A) Metachromatic leukodystrophy
(B) Multifocal leukoencephalopathy
(C) Guillain-Barré syndrome
(D) Hypoxic encephalopathy
(E) Hypertensive encephalopathy

398. Which of the following tumors is characterized by pseudopalisading, necrosis, endoneurial proliferation, hypercellularity, and atypical nuclei?

(A) Schwannoma
(B) Medulloblastoma
(C) Oligodendroglioma
(D) Glioblastoma multiforme
(E) Ependymoma

399. A young patient is found comatose in an automobile with the windows up and the engine running. Death ensues within 3 days and an autopsy is performed. Sections through the brain would show

(A) subdural hematoma
(B) epidural hematoma
(C) basilar hemorrhage
(D) brainstem hemorrhages
(E) hemorrhages of the lenticular nuclei

400. All the following statements apply to ependymomas EXCEPT that

(A) they are the most common type of intraspinal glioma
(B) they are the most common primary brain tumor in children
(C) patients may present with headache and papilledema
(D) they may require differentiation from choroid plexus papilloma
(E) histologic sections display rosettes

401. The most frequent of all the following intracranial tumors in adults is

(A) ependymoma
(B) medulloblastoma
(C) meningioma
(D) glioma
(E) metastasis

402. Creutzfeldt-Jakob disease displays all the following characteristics EXCEPT

(A) spongiform encephalopathy
(B) rapidly progressive dementia
(C) worldwide incidence of 1 case per 100,000 population
(D) absence of an inflammatory infiltrate
(E) inactivation by hypochlorite solution

403. The form of motor neuron disease in which there is weakness and atrophy of muscles, without corticospinal tract dysfunction, is known as

(A) amyotrophic lateral sclerosis
(B) progressive muscular atrophy
(C) Werdnig-Hoffmann syndrome
(D) primary lateral sclerosis
(E) Charcot-Marie-Tooth disease

404. Cerebral neuroblastomas are known to

(A) be fairly common brain tumors
(B) be most common in intrauterine life
(C) usually form mature ganglion cells
(D) elaborate catecholamines rarely
(E) usually form extraneural metastases

DIRECTIONS: Each question below contains four suggested responses of which **one or more** is correct. Select

A	if	**1, 2, and 3**	are correct
B	if	**1 and 3**	are correct
C	if	**2 and 4**	are correct
D	if	**4**	is correct
E	if	**1, 2, 3, and 4**	are correct

405. True statements about meningiomas include which of the following?

(1) They constitute at least 15 percent of all brain tumors
(2) They are more common in children than in adults
(3) They are more common in women than in men
(4) They usually are not amenable to surgical therapy

406. Transection of a peripheral nerve will result in which of the following?

(1) Dissolution of the Nissl substance in the nerve cell body
(2) Degeneration of the nerve fiber distal to the cut
(3) Proliferation of the Schwann sheath from the proximal nerve segment
(4) Degeneration of the axons from 1 to 3 nodes of Ranvier proximal to the cut

407. Lesions associated with acquired immunodeficiency syndrome (AIDS) include which of the following?

(1) Primary malignant lymphoma of brain
(2) Subacute encephalitis with multinucleate cells
(3) Progressive multifocal leukoencephalopathy
(4) Aseptic meningitis

408. Important causes of cerebral infarction include

(1) arteriosclerotic vascular disease
(2) acute lead poisoning
(3) cerebral embolization
(4) equine encephalitis

409. True statements regarding neuroglial cells include which of the following?

(1) They include astrocytes and oligodendrocytes
(2) They include ependymal cells and microglial cells
(3) All function to shelter and maintain neurons
(4) All function as macrophages, when activated

SUMMARY OF DIRECTIONS

A	B	C	D	E
1, 2, 3 only	1, 3 only	2, 4 only	4 only	All are correct

410. A known alcoholic is brought to the emergency room following an altercation in a local bar. The intern observes respiratory irregularity, coma, and papilledema. Emergency surgery is planned in order to prevent

(1) brainstem herniation
(2) cerebellar herniation
(3) Duret hemorrhages
(4) death of the patient

411. Development of bilirubin encephalopathy depends on the

(1) plasma albumin level
(2) type of hyperbilirubinemia
(3) status of acid-base balance
(4) degree of hyperbilirubinemia

412. A preadolescent male with a history of epilepsy (seizures) and mental slowness has facial skin lesions that have become more prominent in the last several years. On the basis of this information, what other abnormalities have been described?

(1) Cardiac rhabdomyoma
(2) Subependymal gliosis
(3) Renal angiomyolipoma
(4) Periungual fibroma

413. Idiopathic parkinsonism is characterized by which of the following?

(1) Cerebral edema
(2) Depigmentation and loss of neurons in the substantia nigra
(3) Neurofibrillary tangles
(4) Lewy bodies

414. Which of the following tumors may be found arising within the pineal gland?

(1) Pineoblastomas
(2) Embryonal carcinoma
(3) Choriocarcinoma
(4) Craniopharyngioma

415. Diseases that are classified as slow viral infections include

(1) Reye's syndrome
(2) subacute sclerosing panencephalitis
(3) Creutzfeldt-Jakob disease
(4) progressive multifocal leukoencephalopathy

416. Tabes dorsalis causes

(1) bilateral degeneration of dorsal nerve roots
(2) a positive Romberg sign
(3) severe impairment of vibratory sense
(4) progressive sensitivity to pain

417. Of unknown pathogenesis, amyotrophic lateral sclerosis commonly occurs in midlife and

(1) is not always fatal
(2) causes sensory loss secondary to involvement of dorsal nerve roots
(3) produces spasticity of all affected muscles
(4) causes weakness, atrophy, and fasciculations of hand muscles

418. Syringomyelia, once regarded as an inflammatory reaction, is characterized by

(1) softening around the central canal of the cervical spinal cord
(2) loss of pain and temperature senses with segmental distribution
(3) preservation of touch and vibration senses
(4) degeneration extending to the posterior funiculi

419. Subacute combined degeneration

(1) is associated with pernicious anemia
(2) usually affects the gray matter of the spinal cord
(3) causes injury of posterior funiculi
(4) usually does not cause motor impairment

420. Alzheimer's disease is characterized by

(1) dementia
(2) neurofibrillary tangles
(3) diffuse general neuronal loss in the cortex, usually accentuated in the frontal and occipital lobes
(4) senile plaques

SUMMARY OF DIRECTIONS

A	B	C	D	E
1, 2, 3 only	1, 3 only	2, 4 only	4 only	All are correct

421. The lesion shown in the photomicrograph below was removed from a patient's nasal cavity. With no age given and at this low magnification, possible diagnoses include

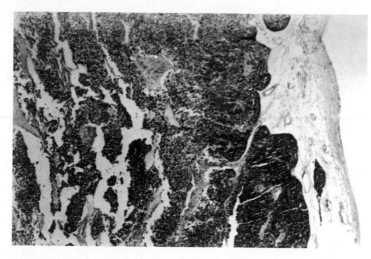

(1) extramedullary plasmacytoma
(2) nasal glioma
(3) olfactory neuroblastoma
(4) nasopharyngeal angiofibroma

DIRECTIONS: Each group of questions below consists of lettered headings followed by a set of numbered items. For each numbered item select the **one** lettered heading with which it is **most** closely associated. Each lettered heading may be used **once, more than once, or not at all.**

Questions 422-426

For each of the conditions below, choose the most appropriate description.

(A) Herniation of the meninges alone
(B) Herniation of meninges and brain parenchyma
(C) Developmental bone defect
(D) Herniation of meninges and a portion of the spinal cord
(E) Herniation at the roof of the mouth

422. Cranium bifidum

423. Meningocele

424. Meningoencephalocele

425. Spina bifida

426. Meningomyelocele

Questions 427-433

For each disease, choose the sign with which it is most likely to be associated.

(A) Accumulation of GM_2 ganglioside
(B) Genetic defect on chromosome 21
(C) Primary CNS demyelination
(D) Abnormal or defective myelin metabolism
(E) Genetic defect on chromosome 4

427. Familial Alzheimer's disease

428. Huntington's disease

429. Multiple sclerosis

430. Krabbe's disease

431. Tay-Sachs disease

432. Metachromatic leukodystrophy

433. Postinfectious encephalomyelitis

Questions 434-439

For each disease, choose the sign with which it is most likely to be associated.

(A) Neurofibrillary tangles
(B) Cowdry A intranuclear inclusions
(C) Optic nerve demyelination
(D) Hepatolenticular degeneration
(E) Verocay bodies

434. Postencephalitic parkinsonism

435. Herpes simplex encephalitis

436. Wilson's disease

437. Pick's disease

438. Schwannoma

439. Devic's syndrome

Nervous System
Answers

389. The answer is E. *(Robbins, ed 4. pp 1405-1406.)* Hypertension is 10 to 20 times more frequent than all the other causes of intracerebral hemorrhage and is also the most common cause of death from cerebrovascular disease. Major sites of hemorrhage, in descending order, are the putamen (more than 50 percent), the cortex and subcortex (15 percent), the thalamus, the pons, and the cerebellum (each approximately 10 percent). Hypertensive hemorrhage shows a predilection for the distribution of the lenticulostriate arteries with small (lacunar) hemorrhages, or large hemorrhages obliterating the corpus striatum, including the putamen and internal capsule. It is possible that development of microaneurysms (Charcot-Bouchard aneurysms) with subsequent rupture is a precipitating factor.

390. The answer is C. *(Robbins, ed 4. pp 1419-1420.)* Astrocytomas are not at all uncommon in the younger age group, but when a child presents with clinical symptoms pointing to the intracranial posterior fossa, a cerebellar medulloblastoma should be suspected, especially if the child has no prior history of leukemia or neuroblastoma. Medulloblastomas occur predominantly in childhood and usually arise in the midline of the cerebellum (the vermis). They do occur (less commonly) in adults, in whom they are more apt to arise in the cerebellar hemispheres in a lateral position. They grow by local invasive growth and may block cerebrospinal fluid circulation (CSF block) by compression of the fourth ventricle. Recent aggressive treatment with the combined modalities of excision, radiotherapy, and chemotherapy have improved survival.

391. The answer is E. *(Anderson, ed 9. pp 2154-2156.)* Smooth-walled cavities in the gray matter are frequent with cryptococcal meningitis, while in tuberculous meningitis solid granulomas may occur in meninges or brain. Subdural effusion is common in *Haemophilus influenzae* meningitis, a common cause of meningitis in early childhood, but is rare in tuberculosis where the exudate is prominent at the base of the brain. Tuberculous infection rarely extends from vertebra to epidural and subdural spaces. In adults it is usually associated with lung disease and in young children with generalized miliary infection. *Mycobacterium tuberculosis* is a strict aerobe and cerebrospinal fluid cultures should never commence with culture tubes upright or horizontal.

392. The answer is A. *(Robbins, ed 4. pp 1416-1417.)* Although several lesions within the brain may be associated with dystrophic or metaplastic calcification, the presence of a calcified tumor-like mass lesion in the cerebral hemispheres should arouse suspicion of oligodendroglioma. Oligodendrogliomas are often slow-growing gliomas composed of round cells with clear cytoplasm ("fried-egg appearance"); they generally occur in the fourth and fifth decades of life. However, some oligodendrogliomas do proliferate in a rapid and aggressive fashion and may be associated with a malignant astrocytoma component. The brown tumor associated with hypercalcemia of hyperparathyroidism is associated with osteitis fibrosa cystica of bone. Some metastatic carcinomas may show microcalcifications in the form of psammoma bodies, as do some meningiomas. Papillary carcinomas of the thyroid and ovary are the best examples of such lesions, but the calcifications found in papillary carcinomas are rarely of the degree and magnitude of those found in some oligodendrogliomas.

393. The answer is D. *(Robbins, ed 4. pp 289-291, 1462-1463.)* Familial cases of retinoblastoma are frequently multiple and bilateral, although like all the sporadic, nonheritable tumors they can also be unifocal and unilateral. Histologically, rosettes of various types are frequent (similar to neuroblastoma and medulloblastoma). There is a good prognosis with early detection and treatment; spontaneous regression occurs rarely. Retinoblastoma belongs to a group of cancers (osteosarcoma, Wilms' tumor, meningioma, rhabdomyosarcoma, uveal melanoma) in which the normal cancer suppressor gene (antioncogene) is inactivated or lost, with resultant malignant change. Retinoblastoma and osteosarcoma arise after loss of the same genetic locus—hereditary mutation in the q14 band of chromosome 13. Probably the normal 13 q14 locus is a suppressor gene.

394. The answer is B. *(Robbins, ed 4. pp 1402-1405.)* Neurons in the central nervous system are most vulnerable to anoxia. The cells affected earliest are those in Sommer's sector of the hippocampus, followed by the Purkinje cells of the cerebellum. The primary motor areas and receptive areas are relatively spared in contrast to the severe involvement of the association areas.

395. The answer is D. *(Anderson, ed 9. p 2158.)* Pyogenic brain abscesses may have a number of possible sources, but the origin can often be determined from the location and number of abscesses in the brain parenchyma. Isolated lesions in the frontal lobes often arise from extension of sinus infections. In the temporal lobe or cerebellum, an isolated lesion may have the middle ear or mastoid as the primary site. Multiple lesions, especially in the superior aspects of the cerebrum, are seen with hematogenous dissemination, often from lung infection or in association with the lesions of congenital heart disease.

396. The answer is E. *(Anderson, ed 9. pp 2187-2188.)* When blood enters the potential space between the arachnoid and dura, a subdural hematoma forms. Subdural hematomas are most commonly located over the cerebral hemisphere convexities. The traditional explanation for the formation of subdural hematomas has been tearing of the bridging veins that pass from the cortical surface to the superior sagittal sinus. Blood may also leak from lacerated cortical vessels or arachnoidal vessels ruptured by a meningeal tear.

397. The answer is C. *(Robbins ed 4. pp 315, 1444.)* Guillain-Barré (GB) syndrome (acute inflammatory polyradiculoneuropathy) is similar to postinfectious (or postvaccinal) encephalomyelitis in that both cause a process of demyelination and show perivascular infiltrates of lymphoid cells (in the brain and brainstem in encephalomyelitis and in the craniospinal nerve, roots, and ganglia in Guillain-Barré syndrome). In addition, the anterior horn cells in GB syndrome may be degenerative. GB syndrome manifests clinically as lower limb weakness and paralysis with varying sensory disturbances, such as hypesthesiae of the lower limbs. The disease may progress to involvement of the musculature of the upper body, including the muscles of respiration, which can lead to respiratory arrest in the absence of mechanical ventilatory assistance. GB syndrome was identified in some persons who were vaccinated with influenza vaccines during the late 1970s.

398. The answer is D. *(Robbins, ed 4. pp 1414-1417, 1445-1446.)* Schwannomas generally appear as extremely cellular, spindle cell neoplasms, sometimes with metaplastic elements of bone, cartilage, and skeletal muscle. Medulloblastomas occur exclusively in the cerebellum and microscopically are highly cellular with uniform nuclei, scant cytoplasm, and, in about one-third of cases, rosette formation centered by neurofibrillary material. Oligodendrogliomas, which are marked by foci of calcification in 70 percent of cases, commonly show a pattern of uniform cellularity and are composed of round cells with small dark nuclei, clear cytoplasm, and a clearly defined cell membrane. Ependymomas are distinguished by ependymal rosettes, which are duct-like structures with a central lumen around which columnar tumor cells are arranged in a concentric fashion.

399. The answer is E. *(Anderson, ed 9. pp 220-222.)* Incomplete combustion of any carbon fuel will lead to accumulation of carbon monoxide gases. Oxygen deprivation results from the formation of carboxyhemoglobin, which displaces the normal oxyhemoglobin and interferes with oxygen exchange. In addition to small petechial hemorrhages of serosa and white matter of the cerebral hemispheres, patients who have lived for several days following exposure will have gross lesions in the brain that consist of bilateral hemorrhage and necrosis of the globus pallidus and hippocampus.

400. The answer is B. *(Robbins, ed 4. pp 1417-1418.)* Astrocytomas are the most common type of primary brain tumor in children and occur mainly in the cerebellum. Ependymomas often occur in childhood and adolescence, but have been noted at all ages. They form more than 60 percent of intraspinal gliomas, but only about 5 percent of intracranial gliomas. Hydrocephalus can be a complication of intraventricular ependymoma. The papillary intraventricular ependymoma is similar grossly to the choroid plexus papilloma. Microscopically, the diagnostic rosette and pseudorosette formations are seen in the ependymoma, with tumor cells arranged around a central space (rosette) or around a blood vessel (pseudorosette). Blepharoplasts, the basal bodies of cilia, are pathognomonic if present.

401. The answer is D. *(Robbins, ed 4. pp 1414-1422.)* Gliomas are the most frequent intracranial tumors of adults; they constitute 40 to 50 percent of such tumors, with glioblastoma multiforme making up 25 to 30 percent. Gliomas at the opposite end of the spectrum include ependymoma and oligodendroglioma, each constituting only 2 to 3 percent. Medulloblastoma also forms 2 to 3 percent of intracranial tumors in adults. Astrocytomas have an 8 to 12 percent and meningiomas a 12 to 15 percent intracranial incidence. Metastatic tumors have an intracranial incidence of 25 to 30 percent with metastatic carcinoma (lung, breast, kidney, GI) and melanoma being predominant. Metastases are often multiple and demarcated from surrounding brain tissue.

402. The answer is C. *(Robbins, ed 4. pp 1400-1401.)* In Creutzfeldt-Jakob disease there is a spongiform change in the cortical gray matter and, sometimes, the basal ganglia are affected. There is little, or no, gross atrophy of the brain and no inflammatory response in brain tissue. The disease is similar to kuru in humans and scrapie in sheep and goats. Rapidly progressive dementia occurs. Worldwide incidence is about one case per million population. The disease is caused by transmissible agents, or prions, which are proteinaceous infective particles, resistant to formalin and ionizing radiation, but inactivated by autoclaving, hypochlorite solutions (bleach), and alcoholic iodine.

403. The answer is B. *(Robbins, ed 4. pp 1432-1433.)* Motor neuron disease is a progressive disorder of the motor neurons in the cerebral cortex, brainstem, and spinal cord and occurs in different forms, depending on the involvement of one or more of these anatomic sites. In progressive muscular atrophy, there is predominant involvement of anterior horn cells, with remittent weakness and atrophy of muscles but no evidence of the corticospinal tract dysfunction that is a finding in amyotrophic lateral sclerosis. However, the basic pathologic processes of these two diseases are similar.

404. The answer is D. *(Robbins, ed 4. pp 1266, 1418.)* The cerebral neuroblastoma is a rare primary malignant brain tumor, usually located in the cerebral hemispheres, and most common during the first 10 years of life. The neuroblastoma is, of course, more frequent in the adrenal medulla, with about 50 percent of neuroblastomas originating in the adrenal and most of the remainder in association with the sympathetic chain. In the cerebral neuroblastoma occasional maturation toward ganglion cells occurs, as in medulloblastoma and in the neuroblastoma of the adrenal medulla, and catecholamines are rarely elaborated, in contrast to the adrenal neuroblastoma. Dissemination of the cerebral neuroblastoma may occur by way of the CSF, as in medulloblastoma. Rare extraneural metastases may develop. Histologically, rosettes and pseudorosettes may be found, as in medulloblastoma and adrenal neuroblastoma.

405. The answer is B (1, 3). *(Robbins, ed 4. pp 1420-1421.)* Meningiomas are more common in adults than in children and occur nearly twice as often in women as in men. The tumors apparently arise from fibroblastic elements normally found in arachnoidal tissue. Because meningiomas occur outside the brain parenchyma and grow slowly, they are uniquely amenable to surgical treatment. Meningiomas are typically discrete and encapsulated, so that symptoms occur as the growing tumor displaces and compresses normal brain parenchyma.

406. The answer is E (all). *(Robbins, ed 4. pp 1442-1443.)* The axonal reaction that occurs when a peripheral nerve is cut includes a number of striking changes. In the cell body, swelling and dissolution of the Nissl substance are apparent within 24 to 48 hours after transection. The axon and covering myelin or Schwann sheath distal to the lesion first degenerate and undergo resorption. In addition, the axis cylinder and Schwann sheath degenerate proximal to the cut over the distance of a few nodal segments. Regeneration occurs when the Schwann cells proliferate from the proximal portion to form a hollow myelin sheath through which the axons grow again.

407. The answer is E (all). *(Anderson, ed 9. pp 2163-2164. Robbins, ed 4. pp 1398-1399.)* AIDS presents a major defect of the cell-mediated immune system, occurrence of many opportunistic infections, and development of unusual tumors including Kaposi's sarcoma, cloacogenic carcinoma, and malignant lymphoma often involving head and neck regions and, occasionally, limited to the central nervous system or the liver. The neoplasm, often of large-cell type, is comparable to lymphoma in immunosuppressed renal-transplant patients. Formerly, it was called *microglioma*. Progressive multifocal leukoencephalopathy (PML) is an opportunistic viral infection of the central nervous system characterized by multiple foci of demyelination. It affects patients with altered immunological states, such as lymphoproliferative disorders, and has been reported in patients with AIDS. Etiologic agents are the papovaviruses JC and SV 40 (-PML). Subacute encephalitis with multinucleate, often giant cells is considered pathognomonic of HIV-1 encephalitis. It occurs in cerebral white matter and cord, and HIV-1 has been found in its macrophages and multinucleate cells. The AIDS dementia complex correlates with this lesion. An aseptic meningitis like viral meningitis occurs in 10 percent of AIDS patients and HIV has been isolated from CSF in some of these.

408. The answer is B (1, 3). *(Robbins, ed 4. pp 1403-1405.)* The major causes of cerebral infarction are cerebral arteriosclerosis, cerebral arteritis, and cerebral embolism. In arteriosclerotic vascular disease, thrombi may form on atheromatous plaques or in stenotic regions. Emboli to cerebral vessels come chiefly from the heart, either from thrombi formed in the fibrillating left atrium, from mural thrombi overlying a myocardial infarct, or from valvular material associated with endocarditis.

409. The answer is A (1, 2, 3). *(Robbins, ed 4. pp 1387-1388.)* The neuroglial cells—astrocytes, oligodendrocytes, ependymal cells, and microglial cells—provide supportive and protective functions for neurons. However, only microglial cells are phagocytic and, in response to injury or destruction of the brain, become activated as macrophages (gitter cells, compound granular corpuscles). Astrocytes support neurons and react to CNS injury by formation of glial scars (gliosis). Oligodendrocytes produce and maintain CNS myelin, and diseases affecting them include multiple sclerosis and the leukodystrophies. The lining ependymal cells do not produce or absorb cerebrospinal fluid. Cell processes of astrocytes, or "glial" fibers, contain vimentin and glial fibrillary acidic protein (GFAP).

410. The answer is E (all). *(Robbins, ed 4. pp 1389-1390, 1409-1411.)* The clinical constellation of altered sensorium and papilledema should call to mind the presence of intracranial pressure, regardless of the cause, which can be due to cerebral edema, tumor mass, or, more commonly, intracranial bleeding with hematoma formation. If the pressure is severe enough, downward displacement of the cerebellar tonsils into the foramen magnum may occur, producing further compression on the brainstem with consequent hemorrhage into the pons and midbrain (Duret hemorrhages). This is nearly always associated with death, since the vital centers, including respiratory control, are located in these regions. Subdural as well as epidural hemorrhages are sufficient to cause critical downward displacement of the cerebellar tonsils. The situation can be remedied with appropriate neurosurgical intervention. In this situation, the downward displacement could be due to hemorrhage-hematoma formation into the posterior intracranial fossa, caused by either a direct (coup) or an indirect (contracoup) blow to the occiput.

411. The answer is E (all). *(Anderson, ed 9. pp 2145-2146.)* Kernicterus is a neurologic complication of severe, unconjugated hyperbilirubinemia that may develop in a jaundiced newborn. Normally, the binding of unconjugated bilirubin by albumin restricts pigment diffusion into tissue cells. However, when the unconjugated bilirubin concentration exceeds the albumin-binding capacity, the lipid-soluble, unconjugated bilirubin is free to diffuse through the blood-brain barrier. Depression of the plasma albumin level; administration of drugs that bind to albumin, displacing bilirubin; and metabolic acidosis all predispose to kernicterus. The bile pigments are noted to discolor the globi pallidi, subthalamic nuclei, hippocampi, dentate nuclei, and inferior olivary nuclei most commonly.

412. The answer is E (all). *(Robbins, ed 4. p 1441.)* Tuberous sclerosis is an important autosomal, dominantly inherited disorder characterized by the triad of epilepsy, mental retardation, and skin lesions. The skin lesions are protean, appear unrelated histologically, and consist of multiple angiofibromas (misnamed "adeno-sebaceum") over the forehead, eyelids, and cheeks. Other lesions are "ash leaf" spots, shagreen patches on the trunk, and periungual fibromas. Periungual fibromas are very characteristic of the disease, if not almost pathognomonic. Visceral involve-ment may include benign cardiac tumors (rhabdomyoma), angiomyolipoma of the kidney, and a peculiar gliosis occurring around the ventricles of the brain. Because of its unique macroscopic waxy appearance, this unusual gliosis has been called "candle drippings."

413. The answer is C (2, 4). *(Robbins, ed 4. pp 1430-1431.)* The pathology of Parkinson's disease remains controversial as to the significance of the observed lesions. In this disease, there is a reduction of pigment in the substantia nigra and nerve cell loss and degeneration. Nigral cells may show rounded intracytoplasmic inclusions that are termed *Lewy bodies.* A small lenticular nucleus and atrophy of the ansa lenticularis have also been observed.

414. The answer is A (1, 2, 3). *(Robbins, ed 4. pp 1272-1273.)* Primary tumors of the pineal gland are very uncommon but are of interest, especially in view of the mysterious and relatively unknown functions of the pineal gland itself. The gland secretes neurotransmitter substances such as serotonin and dopamine, with the major product being melatonin. Tumors of the pineal gland include germ cell tumors of all types including embryonal carcinoma, choriocarcinoma, teratoma, and various combinations of germinomas. Germ cell tumors may arise extragonadally within the retroperitoneal space and the pineal gland, with the only commonality being that these structures are in the midline. Primary tumors of the pineal gland occur in two forms: the pineoblastoma and the pineocytoma. Pineoblastomas occur in young pa-tients and consist of small tumors having areas of hemorrhage and necrosis with pleomorphic nuclei and frequent mitoses. Pineocytomas occur in older adults and are slow-growing; they are better differentiated and have large rosettes. Cranio-pharyngiomas occur not in the pineal gland but above the pituitary gland in the hypothalamus and are thought to arise from structures related to Rathke's pouch.

415. The answer is C (2, 4.) *(Robbins, ed 4. pp 963-964, 1399-1400.)* Subacute sclerosing panencephalitis (SSPE) is caused by the measles virus following infection early in life. There is a long latent period, protracted course, and high mortality. Histopathologic and electron-microscopic changes include perivascular mononuclear cell infiltrates, extensive neuronal loss, and intranuclear inclusions containing para-myxovirus particles in oligodendrocytes and neurons. The CSF contains oligoclonal immunoglobulins against viral components.

Progressive multifocal leukoencephalopathy (PML) is a viral infection of mye-lin-producing oligodendrocytes and causes primary demyelination. Oligodendroglial nuclei are enlarged and contain inclusion bodies, and bizarre giant astrocytes and foamy macrophages with myelin debris are seen in lesions. Electron microscopy reveals papovavirus particles in oligodendrocyte nuclei. Reye's syndrome occurs within 3 to 5 days of viral infection (influenza, chickenpox) treated with aspirin and is associated with severe or fatal brain edema. Creutzfeldt-Jakob disease, a spongiform encephalopathy, is not considered viral in origin but is transmitted by an unconventional agent.

416. The answer is A (1, 2, 3). *(Robbins, ed 4. p 1394.)* Tabes dorsalis causes bilateral degeneration of dorsal nerve roots and the posterior funiculi. During the early phase of the disease, there are sharp attacks of pain because of irritation of the dorsal nerve roots, but later there is a progressive loss of sensitivity to pain, vibration, and proprioceptive stimuli. The interruption of the stretch reflex may result in a positive Romberg sign. The pathogenesis of tabes dorsalis is controversial. Etiologic postulates include focal leptomeningeal inflammation of the dorsal roots, such factors as changes in the structure of the dorsal root ganglia, and a toxic product or metabolic disorder rather than tissue infestation by *Treponema*.

417. The answer is D (4). *(Robbins, ed 4. pp 1432-1433.)* Amyotrophic lateral sclerosis is a disease of unknown cause that may have a prolonged course but is eventually fatal. Destruction of motor neurons occurs in the anterior gray horns, together with bilateral degeneration of the pyramidal tracts, and thus the clinical deficit is mixed upper and lower motor neuron disease. Weakness, atrophy, and fasciculations occur in some muscles, usually in the hands, and spasticity and hyperreflexia in others, usually in the legs. Amyotrophic lateral sclerosis, progressive spinal muscular atrophy, and progressive bulbar palsy differ from one another only in the distribution of the lesions.

418. The answer is A (1, 2, 3). *(Robbins, ed 4. p 1441.)* Syringomyelia is a disease in which there is softening and cavitation around the central canal of the spinal cord. The lateral spinothalamic tracts are interrupted as they cross ventral to the canal; the resultant sensory dissociation involves loss of pain and temperature sense in a segmental distribution but preservation of touch and vibration senses. The cause of syringomyelia remains unknown. At autopsy, the spinal cord is found to contain a cyst surrounded by scar tissue and filled with fluid. The overlying leptomeninges are often thickened. The extent of spinal cord degeneration depends on the size of the cyst and the amount of resulting gliosis.

419. The answer is B (1, 3). *(Robbins, ed 4. pp 684, 1434.)* Subacute combined degeneration is a disease often associated with pernicious anemia or with other nutritional disturbances. The posterior funiculi and pyramidal tracts undergo degeneration, but the gray matter is only rarely affected. Motor weakness with spasticity is the characteristic result. The degeneration is clearly related to B_{12} deficiency, as partial correction of the associated megaloblastic anemia with folic acid does not improve the myelopathy.

420. The answer is E (all). *(Robbins, ed 4. pp 1426-1429.)* Alzheimer's disease is said to be the major cause of organic mental change in elderly patients. If the syndrome of parenchymal lesions of cortical atrophy, neuronal loss, neurofibrillar degeneration, and senile plaques occurs earlier in life, the resultant clinical picture is termed *presenile dementia*. Progression usually results in complete dementia.

421. The answer is B (1, 3). *(Anderson, ed 9. pp 1082, 1089.)* The photomicrograph (at low magnification) shows an intact overlying mucosa with a subjacent highly cellular neoplasm composed of small dark-staining cells ("tumor of small blue cells"). In the child, small blue cell tumors comprise lymphoma, neuroblastoma, cerebellar medulloblastoma, undifferentiated nephroblastoma (Wilms' tumor), retinoblastoma, embryonal rhabdomyosarcoma, and Ewing's sarcoma. In the adult, anaplastic, small-cell carcinomas of the lung, pancreas, uterine cervix, and anorectum (cloacogenic carcinoma); plasmacytomas; and neuroectodermal tumors of thoracopulmonary origin are also included. In addition to the age of the patient and the organ site, certain structures visible at higher magnification, such as rosettes (retinoblastoma) and pseudorosettes (anaplastic small-cell carcinoma, neuroblastoma) aid in the differential diagnosis. In the example given, the lesion is too cellular to be either nasal glioma (large, pale glial cells) or nasopharyngeal angiofibroma (vascular structures). The olfactory neuroblastoma (the tumor depicted in the photomicrograph) arises from the olfactory placode of the stem cell referred to as the *esthesioneuroblast*. The cells populating the tumor are round or oval neuroepithelial cells occurring in clusters and associated with a fibrillary intercellular matrix.

422-426. The answers are: 422-C, 423-A, 424-B, 425-C, 426-D. *(Robbins, ed 4. pp 1438-1439.)* Developmental anomalies of the central nervous system occur under genetic and environmental influences or sporadically during a critical phase in gestation. Various trisomies are examples of genetic mishaps. Environmental factors include drugs (both therapeutic and illegal), ionizing radiation, infections (rubella, syphilis, toxoplasmosis), malnutrition, and circulatory insufficiency.

When the bony spinal cord fails to close, multiple errors, occurring sporadically as single entities or in association with other central nervous system anomalies, are possible. Spina bifida, the most common developmental defect that occurs in the neural tube, involves the failure of the vertebral arches to close completely. Meningomyelocele is herniation of part of the spinal cord tissue and the meninges through such a defect. In spina bifida occulta the defect in the closure of the neural tube is covered by skin and dermis, with only a pinpoint sinus or hair-covered depression marking the site. Bacterial meningitis, or meningomyelitis, is the major potential risk in these patients.

A developmental defect in the skull bones similar to spina bifida is cranium bifidum, which is regarded as a congenital cranial cleft. Meningocele is herniation of the meninges alone through a cranium bifidum.

Meningoencephalocele includes herniation of meninges and brain substance in the region of the occipital bone. Meningoencephalocystocele, a herniation at the roof of the mouth, together with cranial meningocele and cranial meningoencephalocele, occurs less frequently than the herniations associated with spina bifida.

The Arnold-Chiari malformation consists of herniation of the cerebellum and fourth ventricle into the foramen magnum, skull base flattening, and cerebral aqueduct stenosis with hydrocephalus and meningomyelocele. Various combinations of the above abnormalities exist, and it is not necessary for all of them to be uniformly present for the disease to qualify as Arnold-Chiari malformation. In all cases, however, the clinical course is reflected by the degree of hydrocephalus.

427-433. The answers are: 427-B, 428-E, 429-C, 430-D, 431-A, 432-D, 433-C. *(Robbins, ed 4. pp 144-147, 1422-1426, 1429-1430, 1436-1438.)* Tay-Sachs disease (GM_2 gangliosidosis type 1) is one of the lysosomal storage diseases and, more specifically, is one of the sphingolipidoses. Absence of hexosaminidase A leads to accumulation of ganglioside in neurons of the central and autonomic nervous systems and retina. Neurons appear swollen and vacuolated with lysosomes filled with gangliosides. The characteristic cherry-red spot in the macula (due to contrasting gangliosidic retinal pallor) may also be seen in up to 50 percent of cases of Niemann-Pick disease, in which sphingomyelin accumulates.

Major histologic features of Alzheimer's disease include neurofibrillary tangles, neuritic (senile) plaques, amyloid angiopathy, granulovacuolar degeneration, and Hirano bodies. Genetic studies have revealed a genetic defect on chromosome 21 in familial Alzheimer's disease with the gene that codes for the amyloid protein also on chromosome 21, though not in the exact location of the genetic defect of familial Alzheimer's disease.

In primary CNS demyelination there is loss of myelin sheaths, but relative preservation of axons. This type of demyelination is seen predominantly in multiple sclerosis, in the perivenous encephalomyelopathies (acute disseminated encephalomyelitis and acute hemorrhagic leukoencephalitis), and in progressive multifocal leukoencephalopathy. Secondary CNS demyelination occurs because of destruction of the axons themselves.

Multiple sclerosis of unknown etiology causes disseminated but focal plaques of primary demyelination in gray and white matter anywhere in the CNS, but often near the angles of the lateral ventricles. It affects adults between 20 and 40 years of age who may have nystagmus, tremor, dysarthria, paresthesias, and incoordination. A relapsing and remitting course is usual.

In acute disseminated encephalomyelitis (postinfectious or postvaccinial) there are many foci of perivenous demyelination. It occurs, rarely, after a viral infection (measles, mumps, chickenpox) but is not a slow viral infection. Although the disease is fatal in up to 20 percent of cases, prognosis in survivors is quite good.

Abnormal or defective myelin metabolism is characteristic of Krabbe's disease (globoid cell leukodystrophy) and metachromatic leukodystrophy. These leukodystrophies or inborn errors of metabolism usually appear in early childhood. Metachromatic leukodystrophy is an autosomal recessive disorder of sphingomyelin metabolism and results from deficiency of cerebroside sulfatase (aryl-sulfatase A). Sulfatides accumulate in lysosomes and stain metachromatically with cresyl violet. Diagnostic measures include amniocentesis, enzyme analysis, and measuring decreased urinary aryl-sulfatase A. Demyelination is widespread in the cerebrum and peripheral nervous system. Krabbe's disease, also autosomal recessive, is marked by accumulation of galactocerebroside, demyelination, and multinucleate histiocytes (globoid cells) in the white matter.

Huntington's disease is autosomal dominant with its defective gene on chromosome 4. It involves the extrapyramidal system and causes atrophy of the caudate nuclei and putamen. Choreiform movements and progressive dementia seldom appear before age 30.

434-439. The answers are: 434-A, 435-B, 436-D, 437-A, 438-E, 439-C. (*Braunwald, ed 11. p 1997. Robbins, ed 4. pp 956, 1397, 1425, 1431, 1445-1446.*) Postencephalitic parkinsonism (von Economo's disease), one of the complications of encephalitis lethargica, is similar to classic Parkinson's disease in degeneration of the striatonigral pathway with diminished dopamine and depigmentation in the corpus striatum. However, it occurs earlier and is not progressive. In postencephalitic parkinsonism, neurofibrillary tangles, which are thickened and tortuous neurofilaments stainable by silver, form within neurons. In Pick's disease, a presenile dementia, neurofibrillary tangles are also demonstrable, but they are fewer than in either Alzheimer's disease or postencephalitic parkinsonism. Pick's disease is a major cortical degenerative disease associated with marked atrophy of frontal lobes and partial temporal lobe atrophy.

Herpes simplex encephalitis presents a high mortality if not treated with vidarabine (adenine arabinoside, ara-A). It causes necrotizing lesions with Cowdry A intranuclear inclusions in oligodendroglia and occasional neurons. Perivascular mononuclear infiltrates occur and hemorrhagic necrosis is present in the temporal and frontal lobes, especially the orbital gyri.

Wilson's disease (hepatolenticular degeneration) is inherited as a primary defect in copper metabolism with increased copper in liver (cirrhosis) and brain (cavitations). Degenerative cavitations or brown discoloration occurs mainly in the lenticular nucleus and thalamus, and copper pigmentation in the cornea (Kayser-Fleischer rings) is distinctive.

Schwannomas (neurilemmomas) are single, encapsulated tumors of nerve sheaths, usually benign, occurring on peripheral, spinal, or cranial nerves. The acoustic neuroma is one example. Microscopically, Verocay bodies, which are foci of palisaded nuclei, may be found in the more cellular (Antoni A) tissue.

Devic's syndrome (neuromyelitis optica) is a variant of multiple sclerosis with rapid onset of demyelination of the optic nerve and of the spinal cord with paraplegia. A pleocytosis with polymorphonuclear cells and a protein content higher than is usual in multiple sclerosis may be seen in cerebrospinal fluid.

Musculoskeletal System

DIRECTIONS: Each question below contains five suggested responses. Select the **one best** response to each question.

440. The most common tumor that involves bone is

(A) a metastatic tumor from an extraosseous site
(B) osteogenic sarcoma
(C) multiple myeloma
(D) chondrosarcoma
(E) a giant-cell tumor

441. Tuberculous spondylitis (Pott's disease) is characterized by all the following EXCEPT

(A) involvement of thoracic and lumbar vertebrae
(B) hematogenous spread
(C) proliferative synovitis with pannus
(D) destruction of intervertebral disks
(E) formation of psoas abscess

442. The part of a long bone initially involved in hematogenous osteomyelitis is the

(A) metaphyseal region
(B) diaphysis
(C) epiphysis
(D) area around the entrance of the nutrient artery
(E) medullary cavity

443. All the following statements about chondrosarcoma are true EXCEPT that

(A) it is most frequent in middle age or later
(B) the peripheral type can arise from enchondroma
(C) it is common in the pelvic bones
(D) histologic analysis is of prognostic significance
(E) it is the second most common malignant bone tumor

444. All the following diseases may be associated with the grossly deformed joint depicted in the photograph below EXCEPT

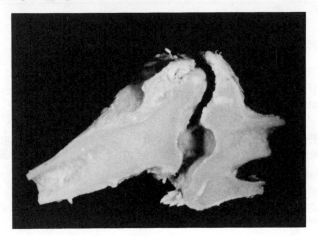

(A) leprosy
(B) psoriasis
(C) syringomyelia
(D) pernicious anemia
(E) diabetes mellitus

445. The lesion illustrated in the photomicrograph below is most likely

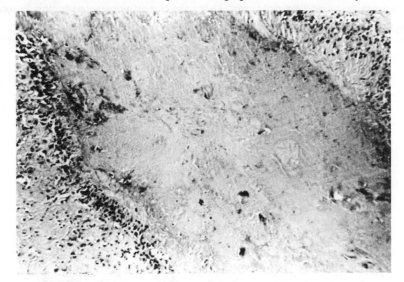

(A) a rheumatoid nodule
(B) myositis ossificans
(C) necrotizing panniculitis
(D) polymyositis
(E) fat necrosis

---

446. Bilateral segmental osteonecrosis or avascular necrosis (AVN) of the femoral head is most often associated with

(A) systemic steroid therapy
(B) irradiation therapy
(C) sickle cell disease
(D) alcoholism
(E) fracture of the femoral neck

447. Osteogenesis imperfecta type I is characterized by

(A) a hereditary defect in osteoclast function
(B) defective synthesis of type II collagen
(C) defective synthesis of osteoid matrix
(D) early death
(E) bone marrow aplasia

448. The specimen shown in the photomicrograph below is from a mass removed from the thigh of a 58-year-old man. Using the current nomenclature, this lesion is compatible with

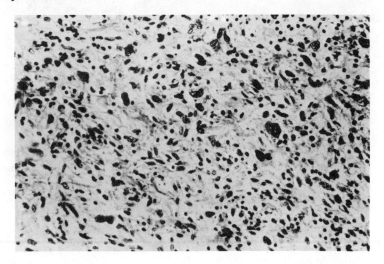

(A) nodular fasciitis
(B) rhabdomyosarcoma
(C) myositis ossificans
(D) osteogenic sarcoma
(E) malignant fibrous histiocytoma

---

449. Which of the following fibro-osseous bone disorders is most likely to be associated with skin lesions?

(A) Osteoid osteoma
(B) Albright's syndrome
(C) Nonossifying fibroma
(D) Polyostotic fibrous dysplasia
(E) Monostotic fibrous dysplasia

450. A sex-linked recessive mode of inheritance exists in

(A) myotonic dystrophy
(B) limb-girdle dystrophy
(C) facioscapulohumeral dystrophy
(D) Duchenne's muscular dystrophy
(E) polymyositis

451. The bone disease shown below in the photomicrograph of a bone biopsy is associated with all the following EXCEPT

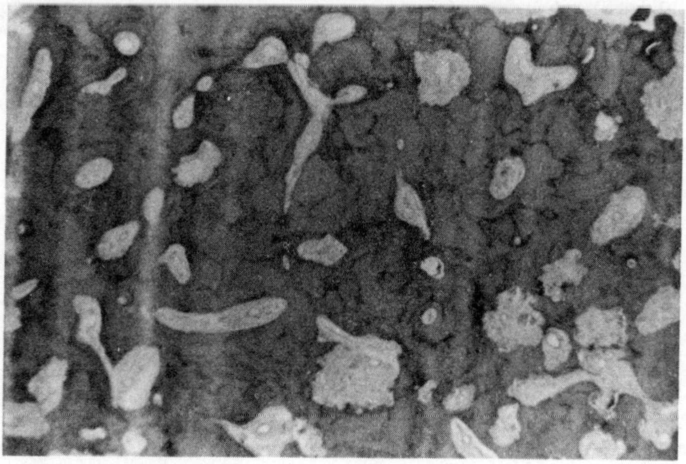

(A) excessive bone resorption
(B) high serum levels of alkaline phosphatase
(C) elevated serum levels of calcium
(D) polyostotic occurrence
(E) pathologic fractures

452. A perivascular inflammatory infiltrate in skeletal muscle, as shown in the photomicrograph below, is likely to be seen in all the following EXCEPT

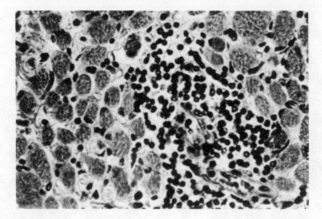

(A) hypersensitivity angiitis
(B) polymyositis
(C) polyarteritis nodosa
(D) cystic medial necrosis
(E) systemic sclerosis

453. The atypical rhabdomyoblasts illustrated in the photomicrograph below may be seen in all the following lesions EXCEPT

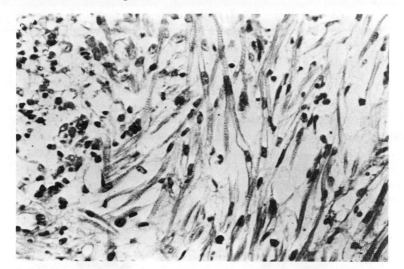

(A) sarcoma botryoides
(B) myositis ossificans
(C) mixed heterologous müllerian tumor of the uterus
(D) adult pleomorphic rhabdomyosarcoma
(E) embryonal rhabdomyosarcoma

DIRECTIONS: Each question below contains four suggested responses of which **one or more** is correct. Select

A	if	**1, 2, and 3**	are correct
B	if	**1 and 3**	are correct
C	if	**2 and 4**	are correct
D	if	**4**	is correct
E	if	**1, 2, 3, and 4**	are correct

454. In the radiograph reproduced in the photograph below, the juxtacortical (parosteal) osteosarcoma shown arising in the distal tibia

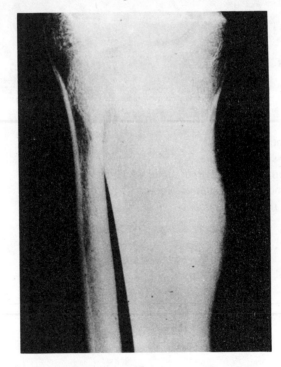

(1) may be confused with myositis ossificans
(2) is primarily composed of cartilage
(3) has a much better prognosis than osteosarcoma arising within the bone shaft
(4) is usually secondary to trauma

455. Osteogenic sarcoma, shown below in a photograph of an x-ray of a hemisected tibia,

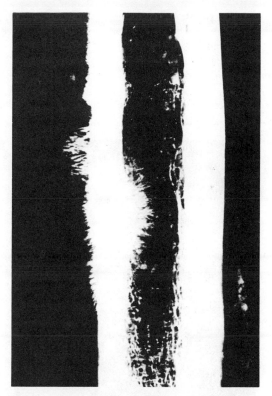

(1) is the most common type of bone cancer in the young
(2) may be associated with Paget's disease in the elderly
(3) features calcified perpendicular striae of reactive periosteum
(4) has a 5-year survival rate of 30 percent with combined therapy

456. Giant-cell tumors of bone (osteo-clastomas) are known to

(1) occur rarely under the age of 15
(2) occur commonly around the knee
(3) show unpredictable biologic behavior
(4) arise in the epiphyseal ends of long bones

SUMMARY OF DIRECTIONS

A	B	C	D	E
1, 2, 3 only	1, 3 only	2, 4 only	4 only	All are correct

457. Multiple, focal osteolytic lesions in the skull, as shown in the x-ray photograph below, are usually associated with

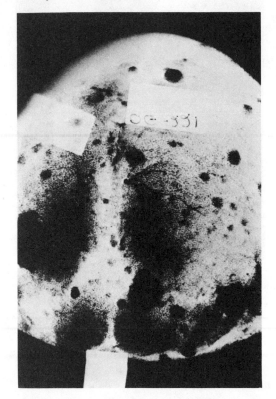

(1) increased production of monoclonal immunoglobulin
(2) prostatic carcinoma
(3) proliferation of neoplastic plasma cells
(4) Ewing's tumor

DIRECTIONS: Each group of questions below consists of lettered headings followed by a set of numbered items. For each numbered item select the **one** lettered heading with which it is **most** closely associated. Each lettered heading may be used **once, more than once, or not at all.**

Questions 458-461

For each disease choose the artist's representation of a microradiogram, shown below, with which it is most likely to be associated. Answer "E" if the disease is not associated with any of the microradiograms.

A   B

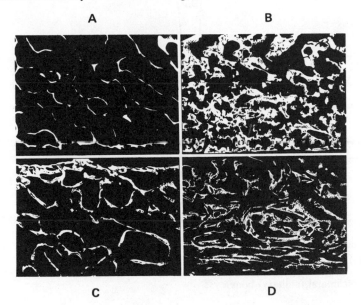

C   D

E None of the above

458. Primary hyperparathyroidism

459. Vitamin D–resistant rickets

460. Osteoporosis

461. Paget's disease

Questions 462-466

For each bone lesion, select the lettered location and general configuration with which it is most likely to be associated in the diagram below.

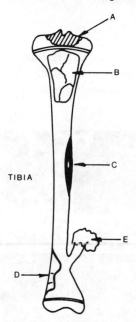

462. Giant-cell tumor of bone (osteo-clastoma)

463. Unicameral (solitary) bone cyst

464. Osteochondroma

465. Osteoid-osteoma

466. Nonossifying fibroma of bone

DIRECTIONS: The group of questions below consists of four lettered headings followed by a set of numbered items. For each numbered item select

A	if the item is associated with	(A) **only**
B	if the item is associated with	(B) **only**
C	if the item is associated with	**both** (A) and (B)
D	if the item is associated with	**neither** (A) nor (B)

Each lettered heading may be used **once, more than once, or not at all.**

Questions 467-470

(A) Ewing's sarcoma of bone
(B) Osteogenic sarcoma
(C) Both
(D) Neither

467. Peak incidence at ages 10 to 20

468. Glycogen-positive tumor cells on PAS staining

469. No significant radiographic findings

470. Prior irradiation

Musculoskeletal System
Answers

440. The answer is A. *(Anderson, ed 9. pp 2055-2056.)* Metastases account for the majority of bone tumors, followed in frequency by multiple myeloma and osteogenic sarcoma. Common carcinomas that metastasize to bone include lung, thyroid, breast, prostate, and renal cell carcinomas. Whereas most metastatic carcinomas to bone produce osteolytic radiologic lesions, prostate carcinoma tends to produce osteoblastic metastases. The serum calcium and alkaline phosphatase may be elevated in osseous metastases.

441. The answer is C. *(Robbins, ed 4. pp 1322, 1354.)* Pott's disease of the spine is caused by tuberculous infection of the lower thoracic and lumbar vertebrae. Destruction of the intervertebral disks and adjacent vertebral bodies causes them to collapse, and these compression fractures may result in angular kyphosis or scoliosis. Caseous material may extend from the vertebrae into paravertebral muscles and along the psoas muscle sheath to form a psoas abscess in the inguinal regions. Tuberculous osteomyelitis occurs most often in the long bones and spine and via hematogenous spread from a primary site elsewhere. Chronic proliferative synovitis with pannus formation is characteristic of rheumatoid arthritis and Lyme arthritis. In Lyme arthritis there is also hyperplastic "onionskin" arteriolar thickening (similar to that in syphilis).

442. The answer is A. *(Robbins, ed 4. pp 1320-1322.)* Nutrient arteries to long bones divide to supply the metaphyses and diaphyses. In the metaphyses, the arteries become arterioles and finally form capillary loops adjacent to epiphyseal plates. This anatomic feature allows bacteria to settle in the region of the metaphysis and makes it the site initially involved in hematogenous osteomyelitis. As a consequence of vascular and osteoclastic resorption, the infected bone is replaced by fibrous connective tissue. Persistent chronic osteomyelitis is often associated with sequelae that include amyloidosis and the appearance of malignant tumors in old sinus tracts within the damaged bone.

443. The answer is E. *(Robbins, ed 4. pp 1340-1342.)* Chondrosarcoma shows a peak incidence in the sixth and seventh decades. Most chondrosarcomas (85 percent) arise de novo, but the peripheral type, unlike the central type, may arise in benign tumors of cartilage, especially if they are multiple. Frequent sites of origin include pelvic bones (50 percent), humerus, femur, ribs, and spine. Although a fairly common form of bone cancer, chondrosarcoma is preceded in frequency by metastatic carcinoma, multiple myeloma, and osteosarcoma. Histologic grading is most important in prognosis since grade I and grade II lesions present very good 5-year survival rates following surgery, unlike grade III, poorly differentiated tumors, which invade quickly and metastasize to lungs.

444. The answer is B. *(Anderson, ed 9. pp 2068, 2158. Bullough, p 7.16.)* The photograph displays a grossly deformed knee joint, an example of neurogenic arthropathy (Charcot's joint). This is a rapidly destructive, often monarticular form of osteoarthritis. Destruction of the joint surface, subluxation or dislocation, and loose bodies are prominent, and the scarred, chronically inflamed synovium contains striking bone and cartilage detritus. The underlying neurologic lesion with its resultant loss of local proprioception and sensory nerve paths may occur in tabes dorsalis, syringomyelia, leprosy, diabetes, spina bifida, or chronic alcoholism. The rare association of arthritis and psoriasis characteristically affects the distal interphalangeal joints of hands and feet in asymmetric fashion.

445. The answer is A. *(Anderson, ed 9. pp 2079, 2082-2083.)* Rheumatoid arthritis frequently affects the small joints of the hands and feet. The larger joints are involved later. Subcutaneous nodules, with a necrotic focus surrounded by palisades of proliferating cells, are seen in some cases. In the joints, the synovial membrane is thickened by a granulation tissue pannus that is infiltrated by many inflammatory cells. Nodular collections of lymphocytes resembling follicles are characteristically seen. The thickened synovial membrane may develop villous projections, and the joint cartilage is attacked and destroyed.

446. The answer is A. *(Anderson, ed 9. pp 163-164. Bullough, pp 7.2-7.8.)* AVN of bone is a moderately frequent complication of high-dose systemic corticosteroid therapy—the usual cause of bilateral segmental infarction or AVN of the femoral head. Clinical features include sudden onset of severe pain and difficulty in walking, with AVN accounting for about 20 percent of hip diseases requiring prosthetic replacement. Within the femoral head a triangular yellow area of necrotic bone is found beneath the viable articular cartilage, and x-ray may show a crescent sign or space between cartilage and underlying infarct. Fracture of the subcapital femoral neck is frequently associated with unilateral AVN; the other conditions listed are much less frequently associated.

447. The answer is C. *(Bullough, pp 3.2-3.8. Robbins, ed 4. p 1318.)* Osteogenesis imperfecta (OI), or brittle bone disease, constitutes a group of disorders often inherited as autosomal dominant traits and caused by genetic mutations involving the synthesis of type I collagen, which comprises about 90 percent of the osteoid, or bone matrix. Very early perinatal death and multiple fractures occur in OI type II, which is often autosomal recessive. The major variant of OI, type I, is compatible with survival; after the perinatal period fractures occur in addition to other signs of defective collagen synthesis such as thin, translucent, blue sclerae; laxity of joint ligaments; deafness from otosclerosis; and abnormal teeth. A hereditary defect in osteoclast function with decreased bone resorption and bone overgrowth, which sometimes narrows or obliterates the marrow cavity, is characteristic of osteopetrosis, or marble bone disease.

448. The answer is E. *(Anderson, ed 9. pp 1853-1860.) Malignant fibrous histiocytoma (MFH)* is the current term used to designate sarcomatous growths of the deep soft tissues. This is principally a disease of the lower extremity and thigh in middle- to advanced-aged patients of both sexes, but it has also been reported as occurring in far-removed areas, such as the adventitia of the thoracic aorta and the ocular orbit. It has also occurred with some frequency years after irradiation. The tumor is composed of a background of spindle cells with varying amounts of collagen (hence, fibrous) and scattered, giant, bizarre, xanthomatous and myoblastic-like cells (hence, histiocytic). In the past, many of these tumors were undoubtedly labeled as "pleomorphic liposarcomas" and "pleomorphic adult rhabdomyosarcomas," both of which must be differentiated from MFH. This does not imply, of course, that pleomorphic liposarcomas and adult rhabdomyosarcomas do not exist simply because a new term has been introduced, but rather that strict histologic criteria should be adhered to in order to exclude MFH—namely, that unequivocal malignant myoblasts with cytoplasmic striations (rhabdomyosarcoma) and lipoblasts (liposarcoma) must be demonstrated. The prognosis is poor for MFH.

449. The answer is B. *(Robbins, ed 4. pp 1331-1336.)* Fibroosseous lesions of bone classically include fibrous dysplasia (FD), nonossifying fibroma (fibrous cortical defect), and osteoid osteoma. Histologically, FD shows a characteristic "Chinese-lettering" effect of the bony trabeculae, which are surrounded by a cellular, fibrous stroma, with osteoblasts and osteoclasts conspicuously decreased at the periphery of the entrapped woven bone. Histologically, nonossifying fibroma shows characteristic foam cell histiocytes within the lesions of the metaphysis. Osteoid osteomas are found within the diaphysis of long bones and contain osteoid trabeculae in a cellular, fibrous matrix, but unlike FD, this disease demonstrates (singular) peripheral trabecular osteoblasts. FD produces radiolucent bone lesions involving long bones and thorax, skull, and facial bones. *Monostotic FD* refers to single-bone involvement, *polyostotic FD* refers to involvement of multiple lesions or bones, and *Albright's syndrome* refers to polyostotic bone lesions, endocrinopathy (hyperthyroidism, thyrotoxicosis, hyperpituitarism, Cushing's syndrome), precocious puberty in females, and café au lait spots on the skin. The pigmented, macular café au lait spots are usually more irregular ("coast of Maine") in outline than the forms seen in neurofibromatosis. Monostotic FD is very rarely associated with the skin lesions.

450. The answer is D. *(Anderson, ed 9. pp 2111-2112.)* Classification of the muscular dystrophies is based on the mode of inheritance and clinical features.

Inheritance of the Duchenne type is by an X-linked recessive trait, with the gene located on the short arm of the X chromosome, although spontaneous mutations are fairly common. Autosomal dominant inheritance characterizes both myotonic dystrophy and the facioscapulohumeral type, while limb-girdle dystrophy is autosomal recessive. In Duchenne's muscular dystrophy, males are affected and symptoms begin before the age of 4. Pelvic girdle muscles are affected with resultant difficulty in walking, and this is followed by shoulder-girdle weakness and eventual involvement of respiratory and cardiac muscles with death from respiratory failure before age 20. Histologic changes include rounded, atrophic fibers, hypertrophied fibers, degenerative and regenerative changes in adjacent myocytes, and necrotic fibers invaded by histiocytes. Elevation of serum creatine kinase is marked.

451. The answer is C. *(Anderson, ed 9. pp 2006-2011.)* Paget's disease, or osteitis deformans, is characterized by excessive resorption of bone and replacement by abnormally soft, poorly mineralized matrix. Since formation of new bone occurs almost simultaneously, serum levels of calcium are normal. Serum levels of alkaline phosphatase are usually higher than in any other bone disorder. Pathologic fractures are fairly frequent in vertebrae (back pain), tibia, femur, or humerus. Polyostotic occurrence is more usual than monostotic. Histologically, the mosaic pattern of cement lines traversing thick, irregular bone trabeculae is characteristic of the sclerotic, or late, phase of Paget's disease (abnormally hard bone).

452. The answer is D. *(Robbins, ed 4. pp 138, 208-210, 571-574.)* Cystic medial necrosis is not inflammatory, but degenerative. Hypersensitivity angiitis primarily affects small vessels; polyarteritis nodosa affects small to medium-sized arteries. In addition to interstitial inflammation (often perivascular), patients with polymyositis have histologic evidence of muscle fiber death. Perivascular inflammation is one of the early skeletal muscle changes in scleroderma (systemic sclerosis).

453. The answer is B. *(Robbins, ed 4. pp 1373-1377, 1381-1382.)* Myositis ossificans is a benign condition characterized by fibrous repair of a skeletal muscle or subcutaneous fat, hematoma with secondary cartilage formation, ossification, and calcification. The other lesions mentioned are malignant neoplasms that may contain a variety of mesodermal tissues. Many tumors diagnosed as rhabdomyosarcoma in the past would be classified as malignant fibrous histiocytoma today, although if cell striations are present in the cells, the lesions still qualify as rhabdomyosarcoma.

454. The answer is B (1, 3). *(Anderson, ed 9. pp 2032-2034.)* Juxtacortical (parosteal) osteosarcoma, an uncommon variant of osteosarcoma, usually has a less malignant-appearing stroma and may even be confused histologically with a benign condition such as myositis ossificans. Trauma does not usually precede juxtacortical (parosteal) osteosarcoma, which has a better prognosis than osteosarcoma of the shaft or medullary cavity.

455. The answer is A (1, 2, 3). *(Robbins, ed 4. pp 1336-1338.)* The characteristic sunburst shown in the x-ray is due to calcified perpendicular striae of reactive periosteum adjacent to the growing tumor. Osteosarcoma, the most common bone cancer of children, can occur in the elderly, in whom the sarcoma is almost always associated with Paget's disease. With surgery, radiation, and chemotherapy the 5-year survival is now about 60 percent.

456. The answer is E (all). *(Anderson, ed 9. pp 2043-2045.)* Giant-cell tumors of bone arise eccentrically in long-bone epiphyses, most commonly around the knee, in young to middle-aged adults (20 to 55 years) and are rare under 15 years of age. They show unpredictable and variable biologic behavior; even lesions that appear benign may recur following therapy, the overall recurrence rate being 25 to 50 percent. The fibroblast-like, prominent, spindle-cell tumor stroma forms the neoplastic element, and the numerous giant cells with features of osteoclasts, scattered regularly throughout the lesion, do not. Many lesions with numerous giant cells simulate it, but it has definite characteristics—it is grossly hemorrhagic, reddish-brown, and gray with central cystic degeneration and a fairly typical x-ray appearance of a lobulated, lytic lesion within the epiphysis.

457. The answer is B (1, 3). *(Robbins, ed 4. pp 739-743.)* Metastatic lesions from carcinoma of the prostate are usually osteoblastic. Multiple osteolytic skull lesions are characteristic of multiple myeloma. Myeloma tumors typically produce gelatinous regions of osteolysis within the marrow cavities of involved bones. Coalescence of these foci may cause erosion of the cortical bone and occasionally will produce through-and-through defects. Histologic evidence of bone necrosis with new bone formation is very rare in myeloma lesions.

458-461. The answers are: 458-C, 459-D, 460-A, 461-B. *(Anderson, ed 9. pp 1975-1977, 1983-1984, 1993, 2006.)* Primary hyperparathyroidism causes increased size of lacunae in the trabeculae of the bones and is associated with increased levels of parathyroid hormones. Its early lesions consist of loss of calcium and demineralization. For this reason, primary hyperparathyroidism is almost indistinguishable in the early stages from osteomalacia. Osteitis fibrous cystica and "brown tumors" resulting from hyperparathyroidism are very rarely seen today.

Osteoporosis (essential bone loss) causes enlargement of the spaces of bone (the haversian canals) and thus produces a porous appearance in the bones. The loss of bony substance produces a brittleness or softness in the bones. The disease results from either an increased rate of resorption or a decreased rate of bone formation. Osteoporosis can be a manifestation of aging or can be a peripheral effect in a great variety of disorders and other circumstances. These include postmenopause, diabetes mellitus, malnutrition, malabsorption (protein, calcium, vitamin C, and vitamin D deficiencies), Ehlers-Danlos syndrome, Marfan's syndrome, alcohol abuse, heparin administration, methotrexate administration, immobility (such as confinement in bed), and acidosis.

Osteomalacia is demineralization of the osteoid matrix, which results in areas of decreased mineral density and loss of bone rigidity. Rickets is osteomalacia in infants and children. It is usually caused by dietary lack of vitamin D. Osteomalacia in adults is, as it were, vitamin D–resistant rickets. The defect in vitamin D resistance involves a failure of D to be converted to $1,25\text{-}(OH)_2D_3$, which is the metabolically active form of the vitamin. Other examples of this defect are advanced renal disease, or renal osteodystrophy, and congenital absence of 25-hydroxylase.

Paget's disease of bone, or osteitis deformans, is seen late in life. It is a benign disorder of bone characterized by increased skeletal remodeling. The skeletal remodeling is indicated by marked increases both in the amount of resorption activity and in the amount of bone-formation activity. Specifically, there is progressive erosion of cancellous bone spicules, with fibroconnective tissue replacement and eventual concomitant osteoclastic bone resorption with osteoblastic bone formation. A mosaic pattern, caused by persistence of visible osteoid seams, is seen in biopsy material.

462-466. The answers are: 462-A, 463-B, 464-E, 465-C, 466-D. *(Anderson, ed 9. pp 2021-2022, 2043-2045.)* Osteoclastoma, the giant-cell tumor of bone, usually produces a lytic lesion involving the epiphysis of long bones. The proximal tibia is a common site. Unicameral, or solitary, cysts are loculated, lytic lesions of bone that characteristically abut on the epiphyseal plate in older children and produce cortical irregularities. Regions involved in the benign lesion are prone to fracture. Osteochondromas are cauliflower-like lesions that contain a core of cortical and medullary bone and a cartilage cap that decreases in width as age increases. Osteochondromas usually protrude from the metaphyses of long bones and may be multiple. Osteoid-osteomas occur most frequently in the cortex of the diaphysis of long limb bones, particularly the tibia. A small radiolucent nidus is usually surrounded by dense, sclerotic bone. Clinically, the lesion is often associated with pain. Nonossifying fibromas of bone, usually well-demarcated, eccentric, lytic metaphyseal lesions, most commonly occur in the tibia and femur. Nonossifying fibromas of bone are histologically identical to fibrous cortical defects and consist of a fibroblastic growth without concomitant bone formation.

There are many pitfalls involved in making a diagnosis of giant-cell tumor of bone. The main problem involves the difficulty of distinguishing the bone destruction that is a true neoplasm from bone destruction that is the result of various types of osteoclastic-osteoblastic activity. Direct communication with the radiologist and, preferably, the orthopedic surgeon is, therefore, nearly mandatory for the pathologist when making a diagnosis.

467-470. The answers are: 467-C, 468-A, 469-D, 470-B. *(Robbins, ed 4. pp 1336-1339, 1342-1343.)* Both Ewing's and osteogenic sarcomas are primary malignant bone tumors that occur predominantly in children and young adults in the second decade of life. However, osteosarcoma can occur in adults over age 40 who have multifocal Paget's disease, or who have been exposed to bone irradiation or to radium-containing paints. Ewing's sarcoma may occur below the age of 10, but is rare below 3. Ewing's tumor usually exhibits glycogen-positive, diastase-sensitive cytoplasmic granules with PAS staining, and electron microscopy demonstrates glycogen in the tumor cells, which is helpful in differentiation from lymphoma and neuroblastoma. Radiographs in osteosarcoma may show periosteal elevation at an acute angle (Codman's triangle) or tumor penetration of cortical bone with extension into the soft tissues. In Ewing's sarcoma reactive new bone formation, subperiosteal and sequential, may cause concentric "onionskin" layering in half the cases. Osteosarcomas usually arise in the metaphyses of long bones of the extremities (lower end of femur, upper end of tibia, upper end of humerus, and upper femur), although they may involve any bone. The origin of Ewing's sarcoma is often the medullary cavity of long bones, innominate bone, or scapula, but the origin may be any bone in diaphysis or metaphysis.

Prognoses for both osteosarcoma and Ewing's tumor have improved in recent years with the combination of surgery and chemotherapy: a 3-year survival of approximately 70 percent in osteogenic sarcoma of osteoblastic type, and a 5-year survival of nearly 70 percent in Ewing's sarcoma. The telangiectatic and the chondroblastic osteosarcomas do not respond as well. Osteosarcomas show marked variation histologically. The malignant osteoblasts may be small and fairly uniform or highly pleomorphic with bizarre shapes and numerous mitoses. If predominantly composed of small round cells with little tumor osteoid or bone, they can be confused with Ewing's sarcoma.

Skin and Breast

DIRECTIONS: Each question below contains five suggested responses. Select the **one best** response to each question.

471. A 56-year-old woman has for 1 year's duration indurated plaques and nodules about the lower back and proximal thighs; the skin biopsy is seen below. What nuclear features are characteristic for this disorder?

(A) Markedly thickened nuclear membranes
(B) Unusually large nucleoli
(C) Folded, cerebriform nuclei
(D) Numerous mitotic figures
(E) Nuclear pyknosis

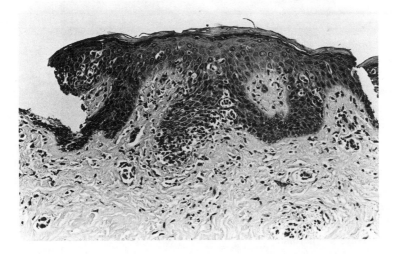

472. A menopausal woman is given a diagnosis of lobular carcinoma of the breast. What impact will this have on her clinical follow-up?

(A) The same impact as other types of carcinoma
(B) The impact depends on node involvement
(C) Biopsies of the contralateral breast are indicated
(D) Radiation should be administered
(E) A tylectomy is sufficient treatment

473. The clinical photograph below suggests that the patient

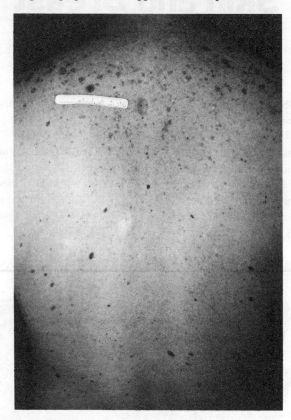

(A) has Leser-Trelat sign
(B) has multiple basal cell nevus syndrome
(C) is at risk for developing malignant melanoma
(D) has leopard syndrome
(E) has Torre's syndrome

474. All the following factors have shown an association with gynecomastia
EXCEPT

(A) Leydig cell tumors
(B) seminomas
(C) Sertoli cell tumors
(D) alcoholic cirrhosis
(E) digitalis therapy

475. All the following malignant tumors of the breast have been known in some instances to have a deceptively bland histologic appearance and hence have at times been misdiagnosed as benign by the pathologist EXCEPT

(A) duct carcinoma
(B) tubular carcinoma
(C) angiosarcoma
(D) papillary carcinoma
(E) metastasizing mucinous carcinoma

476. The most important factor related to the prognosis of breast cancer is

(A) the presence of activated oncogenes
(B) the histologic type and grade
(C) the size of the tumor
(D) the status of axillary lymph nodes
(E) the presence of estrogen receptors

477. An excisional biopsy of the nipple area, taken from a 46-year-old woman, is shown below. The patient complained of discharge from the nipple for approximately 4 months. The most likely diagnosis is

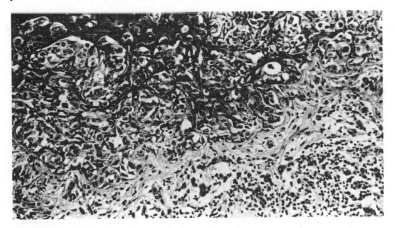

(A) fibroadenoma
(B) epidermoid carcinoma
(C) eczematous inflammation
(D) Paget's disease of the breast
(E) mammary fibromatosis

478. The incidence of malignant melanoma of the skin appears to be increasing in the United States. Which of the following is most significant in predicting the clinical behavior following diagnosis?

(A) The degree of pigmentation
(B) The level and depth
(C) The amount of inflammation
(D) The degree of pleomorphism
(E) The state of nutrition

479. Which of the following statements most accurately describes inflammatory breast cancer?

(A) Inflammation improves the prognosis
(B) Inflammation is increased in Paget's disease
(C) Acute inflammatory cells are present
(D) Chronic inflammatory cells are present
(E) Lymphatic permeation is present

480. Which of the following pairs of disorders would most appropriately be considered in the differential diagnosis for the lesion seen in the photomicrograph below?

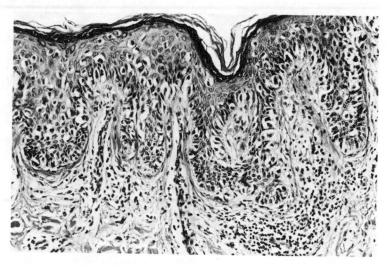

(A) Superficial spreading malignant melanoma in situ and Paget's disease
(B) Mycosis fungoides and metastatic carcinoma
(C) Psoriasis and lichen planus
(D) Lupus erythematosus and lupus vulgaris
(E) Leukemia and lymphoma

481. A 52-year-old woman undergoes a modified radical mastectomy for infiltrating duct carcinoma diagnosed by frozen section. Which of the following statements in the final pathology report is most important in predicting the clinical course in this patient?

(A) The tumor is in the outer quadrant
(B) Two axillary lymph nodes contain carcinoma
(C) One axillary lymph node is 3.0 cm in size
(D) There is apocrine metaplasia in the lower outer quadrant
(E) There is fibrocystic disease in the upper outer quadrant

482. A 37-year-old woman presents with a lump in the upper outer quadrant of the left breast, which shows a wide spectrum of benign breast disease on pathologic examination. Which of the following is considered to indicate the greatest risk for subsequent carcinoma of the breast?

(A) Intraductal papillomatosis
(B) Sclerosing adenosis
(C) Florid papillomatosis
(D) Marked apocrine metaplasia
(E) Epithelial hyperplasia of the ducts

483. A 16-year-old girl undergoes biopsy of a breast lump that shows the changes in the photomicrograph below. What is the most appropriate course of action to follow?

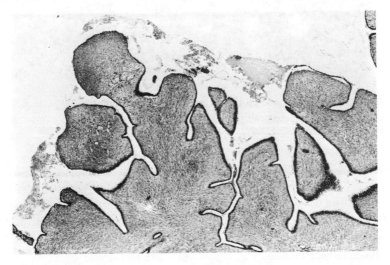

(A) Radiotherapy
(B) Local excision
(C) Radical mastectomy
(D) Modified radical mastectomy
(E) No further therapy

DIRECTIONS: Each question below contains four suggested responses of which **one or more** is correct. Select

A	if	**1, 2, and 3**	are correct
B	if	**1 and 3**	are correct
C	if	**2 and 4**	are correct
D	if	**4**	is correct
E	if	**1, 2, 3, and 4**	are correct

484. True statements about the condition seen in the photomicrograph below include which of the following?

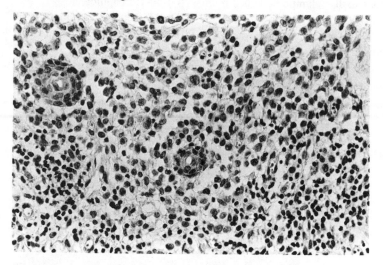

(1) It is often misdiagnosed clinically as seborrheic dermatitis
(2) It may have associated otitis media
(3) It may involve multiple viscera
(4) Birbeck granules can be observed in the cells

485. Malignant or premalignant lesions include

(1) fibrous histiocytoma
(2) senile (actinic) keratosis
(3) keratoacanthoma
(4) Bowen's disease

486. Clinical risk factors for development of carcinoma of the female breast include

(1) late menopause
(2) multiparity
(3) history of endometrial cancer
(4) late menarche

487. An adult patient develops crops of bullae and vesicles in the mouth and later on the skin of the trunk. A skin biopsy is inconclusive but shows a suprabasal acantholysis of the overlying epidermis. Direct immunofluorescence of the skin can be used to identify which of the following?

(1) Bullous pemphigoid
(2) Pemphigus vulgaris
(3) Dermatitis herpetiformis
(4) Erythema multiforme

488. Characteristic histologic features of psoriasis include

(1) parakeratosis
(2) acanthosis
(3) elongation of the rete ridges and dermal papillae
(4) epidermal microabscesses containing polymorphonuclear neutrophilic leukocytes

489. A papillary lesion is seen in a biopsy from a 32-year-old woman who presented with sanguinous discharge from the nipple. Which of the following would be useful in differentiating benign intraductal papilloma from papillary adenocarcinoma?

(1) A cribriform pattern
(2) Knowledge of the presence or absence of cell uniformity
(3) Fibrovascular cores
(4) The age of the patient

SUMMARY OF DIRECTIONS

A	B	C	D	E
1, 2, 3 only	1, 3 only	2, 4 only	4 only	All are correct

490. The differential diagnosis of the lesion depicted below could include

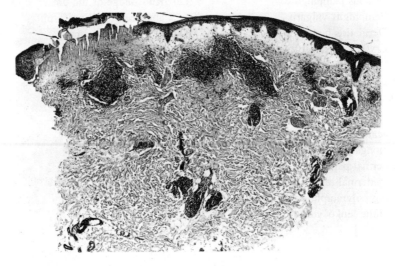

(1) lupus erythematosus
(2) polymorphous light eruption
(3) pseudolymphoma
(4) malignant lymphoma

491. Deficiency of vitamin A might be expected to lead to

(1) mucosal squamous metaplasia
(2) xerophthalmia
(3) follicular hyperkeratosis
(4) night blindness

DIRECTIONS: Each group of questions below consists of lettered headings followed by a set of numbered items. For each numbered item select the **one** lettered heading with which it is **most** closely associated. Each lettered heading may be used **once, more than once, or not at all.**

Questions 492-494

Match the descriptions below with the correct cell.

(A) Merkel's cell
(B) Langerhans' cell
(C) Basal melanocyte
(D) Stratum basale cell
(E) Keratinocyte

492. Has Ia and T6 surface membrane antigens

493. Gives rise to trabecular carcinoma of the skin

494. Receives stage IV melanosomes by a process of endocytosis

Questions 495-497

Match each breast disease with the appropriate description.

(A) Is characteristically painful
(B) May present osteoid or chondroid stromal foci
(C) Is frequently bilateral
(D) Never predisposes to carcinoma
(E) Produces scirrhous tumors

495. Ductal carcinoma

496. Sclerosing adenosis

497. Cystosarcoma phyllodes

DIRECTIONS: The group of questions below consists of four lettered headings followed by a set of numbered items. For each numbered item select

A	if the item is associated with	(A) **only**
B	if the item is associated with	(B) **only**
C	if the item is associated with	**both** (A) and (B)
D	if the item is associated with	**neither** (A) nor (B)

Each lettered heading may be used **once, more than once, or not at all.**

Questions 498-500

(A) Marasmus
(B) Kwashiorkor
(C) Both
(D) Neither

498. Thymic atrophy

499. Dermatoses

500. Inelastic wrinkled skin

Skin and Breast

Answers

471. The answer is C. *(Anderson, ed 9. pp 1469, 1825-1827.)* The characteristic features seen in mycosis fungoides cells consist of folded and enlarged nuclei producing a pattern that has been described as cerebriform or brain-like. At low-power magnification these cells may be missed because of their bland appearance, but at higher magnification the cerebriform, folded appearance is easily seen. *Mycosis fungoides* is actually an older term that is inappropriate in light of current knowledge of this lesion. The cells of mycosis fungoides are a T-cell lymphoma that manifests itself in the skin and that is slowly progressive over many years, pursuing a rather indolent clinical course. A few patients, however, have an accelerated form that can reach a lethal outcome within 1½ to 2 years. The disease is seen in a phase of parapsoriasis en plaque in the skin, which is nondiagnostic as it shows only epidermal acanthosis, and a mild-to-moderate perivascular and band-like infiltrate in the papillary dermis. A very rare mycosis cell may be seen at this stage. The diagnostic stage is when tumor cells are in aggregates in a large packet in the epidermis; this is referred to as a Pautrier abscess.

472. The answer is C. *(Robbins, ed 4. pp 1195, 1198-1199.)* Lobular carcinoma composes up to 10 percent of all histologic types of breast cancer, with duct carcinoma being the most common (70 to 75 percent of the total). It presumably arises from the terminal duct epithelium of the lobule, and it carries a high propensity to multifocality and bilateral breast involvement. There is evidence that this form of breast cancer gives rise to multiple, separate primaries within both breasts. For this reason, breast therapists currently advocate biopsies of the contralateral breast when the tumor is diagnosed. The lobular architectural spectrum begins with lobular hyperplasia and may then progress to lobular neoplasia, atypical lobular neoplasia (lobular carcinoma in situ), and, finally, infiltrating lobular carcinoma. The therapy for lobular hyperplasia and even atypical lobular neoplasia is controversial and is different in various medical centers. If there is any degree of stromal infiltration, however, therapy should at least include a mastectomy; if this is not done, a modified radical mastectomy is required, since the clinical behaviors of infiltrating breast cancers of various histologic subtypes are similar. Some states have written legislation concerning the patient's option to have only excision of the tumor without mastectomy (tylectomy), since more aggressive conventional surgical therapy has not significantly altered total survival over the past 5 or 6 decades. This new approach should be regarded as controversial, however, and more study is needed before the superiority of alternative forms of therapy over more radical surgery is proved. Early diagnosis still remains the best approach to cancer therapy.

473. The answer is C. *(Robbins, ed 4. pp 1280-1284, 1288.)* The clinical photograph depicts the presence of the dysplastic nevus syndrome, first described by Dr. Wallace Clark and his coworkers Drs. Mark Greene, David Elder and E. Bondi in Philadelphia during the mid 1970s. This valuable finding elucidated the presence of abnormal nevi that are at least a marker for the development of malignant melanoma. These nevi, while not malignant, have atypical features compared with those of normal nevi, such as irregular borders, a pink base, and irregular pigmentation. The Leser-Trelat sign refers to the development of multiple seborrheic keratoses over a short period of time in older patients who have visceral malignancy, while the basal cell nevus syndrome is dominantly inherited with the association of numerous basal cell carcinomas forming throughout life, bifid ribs, keratocysts of the mandible, unusual facies, and abnormalities of the central nervous system and reproductive system. A familial occurrence of dysplastic nevus syndrome with basal cell nevus syndrome was elucidated at the 1985 meeting of the International Academy of Pathologists by Elliot Foucar. The leopard syndrome refers to multiple flat lentigines that are not premalignant for melanoma, in addition to cardiac abnormalities and ocular hypertelorism. Recent studies have shown that the dysplastic nevus syndrome is not only familial, but may be sporadic in about 6 percent of the general population. The risk of developing melanoma in the dysplastic nevus familial situation is greatly increased over that in the general population. It has been stated that patients with dysplastic nevi belonging to a kindred with dysplastic nevus and familial malignant melanoma have a 100-fold risk of developing malignant melanoma over their entire lifetime.

474. The answer is B. *(Robbins, ed 4. p 1202.)* Gynecomastia is enlargement of the male breast with marked hyperplasia of duct epithelium and proliferation of periductal connective tissue. No lobular or acinar tissue exists. Gynecomastia often occurs in response to hyperestrinism and may be found with functioning testicular tumors such as Leydig (interstitial) cell or, rarely, Sertoli cell tumors. The major cause of hyperestrinism in the male is cirrhosis because of deficient breakdown of estrogenic substances by the damaged liver. Digitalis therapy occasionally causes gynecomastia, and Klinefelter's syndrome frequently does so because very reduced circulating androgen results in relative hyperestrinism.

475. The answer is A. *(Anderson, ed 9. pp 1741-1745, 1748.)* The most notorious malignant tumor of the breast, presenting a deceptively innocuous histologic and cytologic appearance, is angiosarcoma, with its almost unrecognizable anastomosing clear channels lined by flattened and barely visible endothelial cells. If this combination is seen within unequivocal breast lobules and ducts, the pathologist must suspect angiosarcoma. Well-differentiated adenocarcinoma of the breast (tubular carcinoma) demonstrates a tumor that is rather benign in appearance, with small ducts lined by single and innocuous-appearing epithelial cells. Whereas the primary site of mucinous carcinoma of the breasts (colloid carcinoma), with its "cysts" filled with extracellular mucin and signet-ring cells, presents no problem in diagnosis, biopsies of metastatic lesions will not infrequently show sheets of bland granular cells with pinpoint nuclei resembling granular cell tumor of the skin, a benign lesion. Early intraductal papillary carcinomas have been misdiagnosed at times as benign intraductal papillomas, and the reverse error has also occurred. Infiltrating duct (scirrhous) carcinoma presents no diagnostic problem in either frozen or permanent section analysis for the average pathologist.

476. The answer is D. *(Robbins, ed 4. pp 1193, 1200-1201.)* Carcinoma of the breast still causes about 20 percent of female cancer deaths and is the leading cause of death worldwide in women over 40 years of age. It is difficult to predict survival rate, but the status of the axillary nodes is of major importance since negative nodes suggest 70 to 80 percent 10-year survival. There is a significant decrease in 5-year survival if one to three nodes are positive (only 50 percent), and four or more positive nodes at the time of diagnosis usually mean about 20 percent disease-free survival. Obviously, a large size of involved nodes, invasion of the capsule, and fixation to adjacent tissue adversely affect survival. The histologic type and grade of tumor and its size are important also, but nodal involvement (number and size) is the outstanding factor in prognosis. Unfortunately, more than 20 percent of patients with negative lymph nodes do have recurrences and die within 10 years. Although they are of lesser prognostic importance in breast cancers, high levels of estrogen receptors have a better prognosis than lower levels or none, although the best response to endocrine (antiestrogen) ablation therapy is noted with tumors containing both estrogen and progesterone receptors. Amplified or activated tumor oncogenes, such as the neu-oncogene, may be associated with an aggressive tumor and poor prognosis, but this is not yet proved.

477. The answer is D. *(Fitzpatrick, pp 360-361. Robbins, ed 4. pp 1198-1199.)* The biopsy shows infiltration of the nipple by large cells with clear cytoplasm, which is diagnostic of Paget's disease. These cells are usually found both singly and in small clusters in the epidermis. Paget's disease is always associated with, in fact begins with, an underlying intraductal carcinoma that extends to infiltrate the skin of nipple and areola. Paget cells may resemble the cells of superficial spreading melanoma, but they are PAS-positive diastase-resistant (mucopolysaccharide- or mucin-positive), unlike melanoma cells. Eczematous dermatitis of the nipples is a major differential diagnosis, but is usually bilateral and responds rapidly to topical steroids. Paget's disease should be suspected if "eczema" persists more than 3 weeks with topical therapy. Paget's disease occurs mainly in middle-aged women, but is unusual. In Paget's disease of the vulvar-anal-perineal region, there is very rarely underlying carcinoma. Mammary fibromatosis is a rare, benign, spindle cell lesion affecting women in the third decade. Clinically, it may mimic cancer with retraction or dimpling of skin. It should be treated by local excision with wide margins since there is risk of local recurrence.

478. The answer is B. *(Robbins, ed 4. pp 1282-1283.)* Although malignant melanoma of the skin is not as common as squamous and basal cell carcinoma, it is an exceedingly important and somewhat mysterious tumor owing to its often devastating clinical course and occasionally unpredictable behavior. There appear to be strong immune factors that presumably account for some well-documented remissions, lengthy survival after distant metastasis, and rapid growth in renal transplant patients. However, most patients with this form of cancer pursue a course characterized by eventual distant and visceral metastasis, especially if the histologic type is either nodular or superficial spreading. The subtype called lentigo maligna melanoma, found in the sun-exposed skin of elderly patients, generally has a much more favorable outlook. The most important predictors of outcome are the level of penetration into the subepidermis and reticular dermis (Clark levels I through V: I, in situ; V, invasion of subcutaneous fat) and the actual depth of invasion, measured in millimeters with an ocular micrometer (Breslow depth). The survival at 5 years is 90 percent if the tumor is Clark I or II and 0.76 mm or less in depth, but survival falls to 40 to 48 percent if the tumor is level III or IV and greater than 1.9 mm in depth. While some melanoma cells may show cytologic pleomorphism, many aggressive melanomas exhibit uniformity and blandness. Recent work has shown that melanomas arising in the region of the shoulder, upper trunk, and back in men behave in an aggressive fashion.

479. The answer is E. *(Robbins, ed 4. p 1199.)* Inflammatory breast carcinoma is often misunderstood because of the qualifying adjective "inflammatory." The term does not refer to the presence of inflammatory cells, abscess, or any special histologic type of breast carcinoma; rather, it refers to more of a clinical phenomenon, in that the breast is swollen, erythematous, and indurated and demonstrates a marked increase in warmth. These changes are caused by widespread lymphatic and vascular permeation within the breast itself and in the deep dermis of the overlying skin by breast carcinoma cells. The clinical induration and erythema are presumably related to lymphatic-vascular blockage by tumor cells; if present, these findings mean a worse prognosis for the patient.

480. The answer is A. *(Robbins, ed 4. pp 199-200, 1137, 1293-1294, 1300-1302.)* The photomicrograph was taken from a patient with superficial spreading malignant melanoma in situ; it shows individual cells resembling Paget's disease invading the upper regions of the epidermis. The basement membrane zone is intact and there are lymphocytes in the underlying dermis. Cells with clear cytoplasm and malignant-appearing nuclei such as shown here resemble those of Paget's disease, from which they must be distinguished. Some cells of mycosis fungoides will resemble this, but they occur in nest formations called Pautrier's abscesses. Metastatic carcinoma can produce lesions that resemble malignant melanoma, but these are problems relating to the dermis. Leukemia-lymphoma infiltrates mainly involve the dermis, although the epidermis may become ulcerated and atrophic. Lupus erythematosus and lichen planus produce subepidermal lymphocytic infiltrates with no involvement of the epidermis itself. Psoriasis produces parakeratosis and elongated rete ridges but no abnormal cells in the epidermis.

481. The answer is C. *(Robbins, ed 4. pp 1192-1201.)* It is unfortunate that the outlook for survival in breast cancer in the United States has not improved significantly in the 50 years since the days of Halsted, despite newer techniques of xeromammography and ultrasound, greater public awareness, and attempts at early diagnosis. Perhaps hormonal manipulation based on the presence or absence of estrogen/progesterone receptors on the tumor cells will improve the 5- and 10-year survival rates, but at present the overall survival rate is an unacceptable 50 percent at 5 years. If all axillary lymph nodes are negative for tumor on histopathologic examination in the mastectomy specimen, the survival is an optimistic 80 to 85 percent at 5 years, which dramatically falls to only 30 percent if more than three axillary lymph nodes are involved, if one or more nodes are fixed in the axilla, or if any nodes are greater than 2.5 cm in maximum dimension. Three or fewer positive lymph nodes only slightly correlate with a less favorable course. Recent work has shown that if metastatic breast cancer has grown out and spilled through the lymph node capsule, the prognosis also worsens. Breast cancer continues to be already systemic in at least 30 percent of afflicted patients coming to clinical attention.

482. The answer is E. *(Robbins, ed 4. pp 1187-1191.)* The spectrum of benign breast disease includes fibrocystic disease, which is probably a misnomer; adenosis, both sclerosing and microglandular; intraductal papillomas and papillomatosis; apocrine metaplasia; fibrous stromal hyperplasia; and hyperplasia of the epithelial cells lining the ducts and ductules of the breasts. At one time or another each of the above was considered to be a forerunner of carcinoma; however, with extensive studies in the literature, none of these has been shown to necessarily correlate with a greater risk of developing carcinoma with the exception of epithelial hyperplasia. With any of the features, but especially epithelial hyperplasia, adding a positive family history of breast cancer in a sibling, mother, or maternal aunt markedly increases the risk for developing carcinoma of the breast in the given patient. Owing to the advances and technology of xeromammography, there has been an increased interest in calcifications, which are markers for carcinoma of the breast. These calcifications, however, do not necessarily occur within the cancerous ducts themselves and can be found frequently in either adenosis adjacent to the carcinoma or even in normal breast lobules in the region. Stipple calcification as seen by xeromammography is regarded as an indication for a biopsy of the region by some workers.

483. The answer is B. *(Anderson, ed 9. pp 1730-1731.)* The lesion depicted in the photomicrograph is that of a cellular fibroadenoma, a basically benign neoplasm of the breast. Mueller initially described cystosarcoma phyllodes in 1838 and named it for the resemblance of the lesion to leaves. In older women if the stroma is hypercellular with mitoses and peripheral infiltrative borders, it has the capacity to metastasize. In the adolescent female, cellular stroma of spindle cells, occasional mitoses, such as in this example, may not behave in a malignant fashion as in older women. There is only one documented case of death with dissemination caused by lesions of this type in young girls in the literature. Because most lesions like these behave in a benign fashion, conservative but total excision with a small rim of normal tissue surrounding the lesion is all that is necessary in the adolescent.

484. The answer is E (all). *(Robbins, ed 4. pp 745-746, 1292-1293.)* The photomicrograph demonstrates the presence of Langerhans cells in an infiltrated fashion into the upper dermis and shows the reniform nuclei and crowding characteristic of the disorder previously referred to as a form of histiocytosis-X. These are now known to be disorders of Langerhans cells, which have surface membrane FC receptors and react with antibodies to thymocyte differentiation antigens (CD1) and ultrastructural granules referred to as Birbeck granules. The Letterer-Siwe form arises in children, often in infants, and presents with cutaneous lesions that resemble seborrheic dermatitis (or cradle cap). Often these patients present with fever and otitis media or mastoiditis, which call attention to the disorder. If the disease disseminates it may involve organs of the mononuclear phagocyte system, including the spleen, liver, lymph nodes, bone marrow, and lungs. X-ray lesions are reflected by cystic radiolucent areas that can be seen in the skull, pelvis, and long bones. Patients often have anemia and thrombocytopenia, which can contribute to a terminal outcome owing to infections. The term *Langerhans cell granulomatosis* has been offered as an alternative designation to *histiocytosis-X, Letterer-Siwe form*. Many infants died from the disorder in years past, but with the use of chemotherapy and improvement of underlying hypoimmunity, there has been a reversal of the death rate.

485. The answer is C (2, 4). *(Robbins, ed 4. pp 1285-1288.)* Fibrous histiocytoma (dermatofibroma, sclerosing hemangioma) is a benign dermal tumor of fibroblasts and histiocytes, proliferating in cartwheel or storiform pattern, in which small blood vessels may form a prominent component. Senile (actinic, solar) keratosis is a premalignant skin lesion with focal atypia of keratinocytes of the lower layers of the epidermis. There is often a history of chronic exposure to sun, and there is a high incidence in the southern United States. Other precancerous skin lesions include erythroplasia of Queyrat and the active junctional nevus. Keratoacanthoma, a benign tumor, may resemble squamous cell carcinoma both clinically and histologically, but penetration of the dermis never extends deeper than adjacent hair follicles. The lesion is cup-shaped with central keratin; biopsy or excision excludes squamous carcinoma. Bowen's disease is squamous cell carcinoma of the skin in situ. There is no dermal invasion through the basement membrane. The abnormal squamous cells entirely replace the normal epidermis.

486. The answer is B (1, 3). *(Robbins, ed 4. pp 1192-1193.)* Long and continuous exposure to endogenous estrogens increases the risk of developing breast carcinoma. Therefore, late menopause (after age 50), early menarche (especially before age 13), and nulliparity are all risk factors. Endometrial adenocarcinoma and occasional ovarian cancers are also associated with continuous estrogen stimulation with a resultant higher risk of the development of breast cancer in the same patient. Other factors include Jewish ancestry and obesity—estrogen metabolism is altered in obese women and synthesis of estrone increased. Family history is significant, especially if mother and sister had premenopausal breast cancer, in which case there is an increased risk of 50 times that of controls. A past history of breast cancer, especially of lobular type, means greater risk of contralateral breast carcinoma. Hormonal and genetic factors and obesity are probably the major risk factors.

487. The answer is A (1, 2, 3). *(Robbins, ed 4. pp 1298-1299, 1304-1306.)* Patients of either sex in the fourth to sixth decade who develop oral vesicles followed by disseminated bullae are likely to have pemphigus vulgaris, one of the blistering (bullous) dermatoses. The differential diagnosis in this setting is widespread and can include various forms of erythema multiforme (or Stevens-Johnson syndrome in the young), bullous pemphigoid, and pemphigus vulgaris. Common to most bullous dermatoses is the presence of epidermal cell separation, which produces spaces and clefts (acantholysis) that are visible in ordinary tissue sections and specific to location within the epidermis. The bullae may be subcorneal, intraepidermal, suprabasal, or subepidermal, and multiple diseases can be grouped according to acantholysis location. To categorize the type of disease further, direct immunofluorescence testing can be done on a fresh skin lesion, using antibodies to immunoglobulins, fibrin, and complement. Pemphigus vulgaris shows a characteristic "basket-weave" pattern in the epidermis to IgG, IgA is found at the tips of the dermal papillae in dermatitis herpetiformis, and linear bands of IgG and complement are found in the subepidermal zones in bullous pemphigoid, whereas erythema multiforme has no immunofluorescent pattern.

488. The answer is E (all). *(Fitzpatrick, pp 46-55. Robbins, ed 4. pp 1300-1301.)* All the features mentioned plus edema with clubbing of dermal papillae and dilatation of straight capillaries in the dermal papillae are, taken together, pathognomonic, histologic characteristics of psoriasis. The diagnosis of a lesion as "psoriasiform dermatitis" indicates that some but not all of the six characteristics are present. A partial pattern is nondiagnostic and should not be taken to mean psoriasis, since it is a nonspecific histologic pattern that may be found in other conditions, including exfoliative dermatitis, seborrheic dermatitis, chronic contact dermatitis, and neurodermatitis.

489. The answer is A (1, 2, 3). *(Anderson, ed 9. pp 1731-1732, 1737-1739.)* The histologic distinction between benign, cystic intraductal papillomas of the breast and papillary adenocarcinomas is based on multiple criteria. The age of the patient is not of immense importance, since papillomas occur in both younger and older women. Benign papillomas are structured with a complex arrangement of papillary fronds of fibrovascular stalks, covered by one or (usually) two types of epithelial cells. Papillary carcinomas are usually of one monotonous cell type and have either no fibrovascular stalks or only a few of them. Papillary carcinomas show a uniform growth of similar-appearing cells with enclosed tubular spaces, with the whole arrangement bridging across the entire lumen at times or simply lining the outer rim of the duct (cribriforming). Peripheral invasion of the stroma, if present at all, makes the diagnosis of carcinoma rather certain. There are lesions in which the differentiation is exceedingly difficult, even in the hands of renowned surgical pathologists. Many competent pathologists understandably prefer to defer the diagnosis on all papillary lesions of the breast on frozen section until well-fixed and optimally prepared permanent sections are available.

490. The answer is E (all). *(Anderson, ed 9. pp 1769-1771, 1827.)* Dense lymphocytic infiltration of the skin carries with it a differential diagnosis that includes the five L's: lupus, light, lymphoma, pseudolymphoma, and lymphocytic infiltration of the skin (Jessner). All are characterized by lymphoid hyperplasia of the dermis. Leukemic lymphomas are diagnosed by atypical sheets of lymphoblastic cells with mitoses; lupus erythematosus is characterized by lymphoid infiltration around the follicles and vessels of the dermis. Light eruptions are characterized by a lymphocytic perivascular inflammation on the skin of the face. A difficult differential diagnosis includes lymphocytic infiltration of the skin (Jessner), which often has an increase in dermal mucopolysaccharides that can be demonstrated by alcian blue stains.

491. The answer is E (all). *(Anderson, ed 9. pp 552-553.)* Vitamin A maintains normal skeletal growth, structure and function of specialized epithelium, and formation of retinal pigments. Deficiency of vitamin A leads to squamous metaplasia in trachea, bronchi, renal pelves, and pancreatic ducts. Such metaplastic epithelial lesions are most common in children. Xerophthalmia (conjunctival keratinization) is often diagnostic and occurs in prolonged mild deficiency. A common skin lesion in adults is follicular hyperkeratosis in which papules develop from formation of keratin plugs in sebaceous glands. Night blindness is common in vitamin A deficiency. Visual purple, or rhodopsin, formed in the retina by combination of vitamin A and protein is essential for vision in partial darkness.

492-494. The answers are: 492-B, 493-A, 494-E. *(Robbins, ed 4. pp 1277-1278.)* The skin should be regarded as a biologic unit, unique by function and structure, containing populations of cells with similarities to other organ cells, but having unique properties by location and function.

The Langerhans' cell is a member of the mononuclear phagocyte system that is probably derived from bone marrow stem cells but spends much of its time within the epidermis itself. These fascinating cells are dendritic and have macrophage markers on their surfaces, including HLA-DR(Ia), T6 thymocyte differentiation antigen, and in some cases FC receptors. They function in processing foreign antigens and presenting the antigens to T lymphocytes. They contain unique ultrastructural granules, referred to as Birbeck granules, which may possibly be related to the surface membrane.

Merkel's cells are poorly understood cells in the upper papillary dermis that may function as neurotactile receptors. These cells are characterized ultrastructurally by dense core granules, which are situated in a circumferential manner around the nucleus and which, when neoplastic, give rise to the Merkel's tumor, otherwise referred to as trabecular carcinoma. These tumors may resemble lymphomas of the skin, from which they must be distinguished.

Basal melanocytes are situated in the stratum basale and are derived from the neural crest. They function in melanogenesis because they contain all the enzymes necessary for the production of melanin, including tyrosinase and dihydroxyphenylalanine. Melanocytes are thought to give rise to melanomas as well as differentiation into nevocellular cells of the dermis, which compose the ordinary mole. They are under the influence of hormones including MSH, ACTH, melatonin, and probably growth and sex hormones. Melanocytes contain the four stages of melanin-associated organelles referred to as melanosomes, which can be distinguished by their stages, ranging from stage I (nonmelanized) through stage IV (totally melanized). The melanosomes can be found on the dendrites that extend from the melanocyte and are in contiguity with cells of the epidermis, otherwise known as the keratinocytes. The melanosomes, especially stage III and stage IV, can be transferred from the dendrites of the basal melanocyte directly to the surrounding keratinocyte by endocytosis. In this manner, melanin is transferred from the melanocyte to the squamous cells, especially in response to sunlight (a process referred to as tanning).

The basal cell of the epidermis is the stratum basale cell, which functions in giving rise to keratinocytes.

495-497. The answers are: 495-E, 496-D, 497-B. *(Robbins, ed 4. pp 1188-1189, 1190-1191, 1194-1195.)* Diseases of the breast that are often painful include galactocele, duct ectasia, and fibrocystic disease. Infiltrating ductal carcinoma rarely causes pain but is likely to produce scirrhous tumors causing a firm or hard mass.

Cystosarcoma phyllodes may be either benign or malignant and has a cellular myxoid stroma in which osteoid or chondroid foci may appear. It forms a large, lobulated, and cystic lesion and malignant change is accompanied by rapid increase in size. Metastases occur only in about 15 percent of cases.

Sclerosing adenosis is benign, does not predispose to carcinoma, is often unilateral, and arises in the upper outer quadrant. It displays clinical and histologic features difficult to distinguish from carcinoma.

None of these three lesions tends to be bilateral—unlike both lobular carcinoma and fibrocystic disease.

498-500. The answers are: 498-C, 499-B, 500-A. *(Anderson, ed 9. p 549. Robbins, ed 4. pp 436-438.)* Marasmus is caused by marked deficiency in total caloric intake, including proteins, carbohydrates, lipids, vitamins, and minerals. Kwashiorkor is linked to marked protein deficiency with adequate or high carbohydrate intake. There are sometimes intermediate forms, or combinations, of these two predominantly childhood diseases. In severe kwashiorkor or marasmus thymic atrophy occurs with reduction in number and function of circulating T cells. B-cell function (immunoglobulin production) is also depressed so that these children are highly vulnerable to infections. Dermatoses, characterized by pigment changes and desquamation, are pathognomonic of kwashiorkor. Inelastic wrinkled skin, due to loss of subcutaneous fat, is striking in marasmus.

Bibliography

Anderson WA, Kissane JM (eds): *Pathology*, 9th ed. St. Louis, CV Mosby, 1989.

Braunwald E, et al (eds): *Harrison's Principles of Internal Medicine*, 11th ed. New York, McGraw-Hill, 1987.

Bullough PG, Vigorita VJ: *Atlas of Orthopaedic Pathology: With Clinical and Radiologic Correlations*. New York, Gower Medical Publishing, 1984.

Fitzpatrick TB, et al: *Color Atlas and Synopsis of Clinical Dermatology*. New York, McGraw-Hill, 1983.

Gottlieb MS, et al: UCLA Conference: The acquired immunodeficiency syndrome. *Ann Intern Med* 99:208, 1983.

Graves HCB, et al: Postcoital detection of a male-specific semen protein. *N Engl J Med* 312:338, 1985.

Grizzle WE, Dunlap N: Cushing's syndrome: Diagnosis of the atypical patient. *Arch Pathol Lab Med* 113:727-728, 1989.

Henry JB, et al (eds): *Todd-Sanford-Davidsohn: Clinical Diagnosis and Management by Laboratory Methods*, 17th ed. Philadelphia, WB Saunders, 1984.

Koss LG: *Diagnostic Cytology and Its Histopathologic Bases*, 3rd ed. Philadelphia, JB Lippincott, 1979.

Morris JG, et al: Cholera and other vibrioses in the United States. *N Engl J Med* 312:343, 1985.

Murray HW, et al: Impaired production of lymphokines and immune (gamma) interferon in the acquired immunodeficiency syndrome. *N Engl J Med* 310:883, 1984.

Reichert GM, et al: Special topic review. Autopsy pathology in acquired immune deficiency syndrome. *Am J Pathol* 112:357, 1983.

Richart RM: Causes and management of cervical intraepithelial neoplasia. *Cancer* 60:1951–1959, 1987.

Robbins SL, Cotran RS: *Pathologic Basis of Disease*, 4th ed. Philadelphia, WB Saunders, 1989.

Rosai J: *Ackerman's Surgical Pathology*, 7th ed. St. Louis, CV Mosby, 1989.

Schwarz WB, Wolfe HJ, Pauker SG: Pathology and probabilities: A new approach to interpreting and reporting biopsies. *N Engl J Med* 305:917, 1981.

Stout J, Yu VL, Zuravleff J: Ubiquitousness of *Legionella pneumophila* in the water supply of a hospital with endemic Legionnaire's disease. *N Engl J Med* 306:466, 468, 1982.

Takahashi M: *Color Atlas of Cancer Cytology*, 2nd ed. Tokyo, Igaku-Shoin, 1982.

Tam R: Culture-independent diagnosis of *Chlamydia trachomatis* using monoclonal antibodies. *N Engl J Med* 310:1146, 1984.

Williams WJ, et al: *Hematology*, 4th ed. New York, McGraw-Hill, 1990.

Wintrobe MM, et al: *Clinical Hematology*, 8th ed. Philadelphia, Lea & Febiger, 1981.